DOPPLER ECHOCARDIOGRAPHY

DOPPLER ECHOCARDIOGRAPHY
A PRACTICAL MANUAL

Pravin M. Shah, M.D., F.A.C.C.
Professor of Medicine
UCLA School of Medicine
Chief, Cardiology Division
Wadsworth Veterans Administration Medical Center
Los Angeles, California

Govindan Vijayaraghavan, M.D., D.M. (Cardiology)
Senior Research Associate
Cardiology Division
Wadsworth Veterans Administration Medical Center
UCLA School of Medicine
Los Angeles, California
Associate Professor of Cardiology
University of Kerala
Kerala, India

K. T. Singham, M.B.B.S., F.R.A.C.P., F.A.C.C.
Visiting Scientist
Cardiology Division
Wadsworth Veterans Administration Medical Center
UCLA School of Medicine
Los Angeles, California
Associate Professor of Medicine
University of Malaya
Kuala Lumpur, Malaysia

Contributors:
Mark J. Callahan, M.D.
James B. Seward, M.D.
A. Jamil Tajik, M.D., F.A.C.C.

A WILEY MEDICAL PUBLICATION
JOHN WILEY & SONS
New York • Chichester • Brisbane • Toronto • Singapore

Library of Congress Cataloging in Publication Data

Shah, Pravin M.
    Doppler echocardiography.

    (A Wiley medical publication)
    Bibliography: p.
    Includes index.
    1. Ultrasonic cardiography. 2. Heart—Diseases—
Diagnosis. 3. Doppler effect. I. Vijayaraghavan,
Govindan. II. Singham, K. T. III. Title. IV. Series.
RC683.5.U5S52 1985   616.1'207543   84-21883
ISBN 0-471-80914-4

Printed in the United States of America

10 9 8 7 6 5 4 3 2 1

To our wives,
Anjali Shah,
Nalini Vijayaraghavan,
and
Puvaneswari Singham,
for their patience and understanding,
and to the Cardiology Staff Assistant,
Mrs. Katherine A. Cherry,
for her unfailing loyalty and support

PREFACE

Doppler echocardiography has had a major impact on the clinical practice of diagnostic ultrasound. Although a number of investigators initially explored the use of pulsed Doppler techniques with either M-mode or two-dimensional echocardiographic imaging, it was not until the advent of continuous-wave Doppler echocardiography that precise quantitation became feasible. The field of Doppler echocardiography is rapidly expanding, as can be judged from the ever-increasing number of abstracts presented at national scientific meetings. It is expected that most laboratories in which state-of-the-art diagnostic echocardiography is performed will acquire and use the Doppler techniques. The pulsed and continuous-wave approaches are complementary and, when used together, permit the diagnosis of valvular obstructions or regurgitation and of intracardiac shunts and blood flows. Quantitative evaluations of obstruction to flow and of intracardiac shunts are major contributions of continuous-wave or extended-range pulsed Doppler methods. In addition, the noninvasive estimations of cardiac output are likely to have major uses in patient management.

Doppler Echocardiography: A Practical Manual is offered as a guide for those new to this field as well as those with some basic familiarity. It should be helpful to physicians and technicians alike. The manual purposely avoids a detailed discussion of the physics of the Doppler principle and its applications. It emphasizes practical approaches that are helpful in performing as well as interpreting Doppler results. Ten of the eleven chapters are authored by workers in one laboratory, which provides uniformity of style and easy reading. Chapter 11 on congenital heart disease is contributed by Drs. Callahan, Seward, and Tajik from the Mayo Clinic. These authors draw on their vast experience in echo Doppler imaging of congenital as well as acquired heart disease in patients of all age groups.

It is with great pleasure that we acknowledge the cooperation and assistance of a number of co-workers. Dr. Maylene Wong, Director of the Noninvasive Laboratory; Dr. Chuwa Tei, Senior Research Associate from Kagoshima, Japan; Dr. Jong Bae, Visiting Scientist from Seoul, Korea; and Dr. Eva Herrmann, Visiting Physician from Dusseldorf, West Germany, provided assistance with patient recordings. Mrs. Ah Lin Wong and Ms. Ruth Alejos provided technical assistance. Dr. Chester Boltwood, Dr. Martin Josephson, and Dr. Maylene Wong provided correlative hemodynamic data. The cardiology fellows in training (Drs. Joseph Caplan, Mark Schwab, Kenton Gregory, Daniel Reiders, and David Gee) referred patients for diagnostic evaluations. Mrs. Linda Lieb provided assistance for the preparation of illustrative material. Mrs. Katherine Cherry and Ms. Cindy Ventuleth provided secretarial assistance.

This study was made during Dr. Vijayaraghavan's tenure as an advanced research fellow at UCLA. He was supported in part by an Investigative Group Fellowship Award from the American Heart Association, Los Angeles affiliate. We gratefully acknowledge funding support from the Arthur Dodd Fuller Foundation and continued commitment to cardiovascular research from its president, Mrs. Betty Samuels. The Irex Corporation provided us with the Doppler echocardiography equipment that made it possible to obtain the high-quality images reproduced in this manual. Finally, much of our clinical academic activity would not be possible without the administrative support of senior officials at the West Los Angeles Veterans Administration Medical Center, Wadsworth Division, including Mr. William Anderson, Medical Director; Dr. H. Earl Gordon, Chief of Staff; and Dr. Lawrence R. Freedman, Chief of Medical Service.

Pravin M. Shah
Govindan Vijayaraghavan
K. T. Singham

CONTENTS

DOPPLER
ECHOCARDIOGRAPHY

1

INTRODUCTION TO DOPPLER ECHOCARDIOGRAPHY

Echocardiography has enabled us to visualize the intracardiac structures noninvasively. M-mode and two-dimensional echocardiography together have contributed substantially to our understanding of cardiac physiology in normal and diseased states. The limitation of M-mode technique is mainly the "ice pick" sampling of the heart by the narrow beam of ultrasound. However, when used along with two-dimensional echocardiography, it is possible to make accurate measurements of cardiac chamber dimensions and of indices of contractility and relaxation, as well as estimates of the ejection fraction. However, these techniques, have limited usefulness in diagnosing the presence and severity of valvar regurgitation and the severity of aortic valve stenosis. Movement of a stenosed valve orifice is a function not only of the anatomic severity of narrowing but also of the myocardial function and consequent cardiac output. One can overcome these limitations of echocardiography by measuring the velocity of blood flow and detecting the abnormal direction of blood flow, as well as by identifying areas of turbulent blood flow, by Doppler echocardiography.

Continuous-wave Doppler echocardiography began in 1961 (Franklin et al), when it was used to measure blood flow in the peripheral arteries. It was found to be useful in the diagnosis of peripheral vascular disease, and has subsequently been used for automatic devices to measure blood pressure. Introduction of pulsed Doppler echocardiography facilitated the measurement of blood flow velocity at preselected depths. This capability, when incorporated into a standard M-mode echocardiographic system, could identify patterns of smooth or turbulent blood flow in various cardiac chambers or vessels. However unless the ultrasonic beam was directed parallel to the blood flow, velocity of the blood could not be measured. This problem was overcome by incorporating Doppler echocardiography into the two-dimensional echo imaging systems, which permitted more precise spatial orientation of the Doppler beam and Doppler sample volume. Pulsed Doppler echocardiography was limited in that it could measure blood velocities of only up to 1.7 meters per second (m/sec). This problem has been partly overcome by newer equipment, in which extended pulsed Doppler technique or continuous-wave Doppler facilities are available along with the conventional pulsed Doppler system. Most of the new generation of two-dimensional echo Doppler equipment is able to measure blood flow velocities in various cardiac chambers or great vessels in excess of 5 m/sec.

DOPPLER EFFECT AND DOPPLER ECHOCARDIOGRAPHY

Christian Johann Doppler (1803–1853) demonstrated that the frequency of sound reflected from an object is altered if that object is moving. A person hears a higher-pitched note if the sound source is moving toward him and a lower-pitched note if it is moving away from him. This change or shift of frequency in relation to the direction of movement of its source is called the *Doppler effect* (Fig. 1.1). The end result is the same if the observer is moving instead of the source of sound. When ultrasound waves are directed toward the bloodstream, the blood cell movements produce a Doppler shift of ultrasound frequencies. The extent and direction of shift of the ultrasound frequency are related to the velocity and direction of blood flow. Hence, a measure of this Doppler shift of ultrasound frequency permits an estimation of the direction and velocity of the bloodstream.

Ultrasound, like audible sound, consists of acoustic waves, but of higher frequency (>20,000 Hz). Sound waves of 1–10 million cycles per second (MHz) are used in diagnostic echocardiography. The echocardiographic transducers are made of piezoelectric crystals and transmit the ultrasound in short pulses. M-mode echocardiographs have a pulse repetition frequency of 1,000–2,000/sec, and two-dimensional echo instruments use pulses of 3,000–5,000/sec. During the pauses between pulsing, the same transducer acts as the receiver of returning echoes. Doppler echocardiography uses ultrasound of the same frequency as the commercially available echocardiographs. It can also be transmitted continuously to the heart from one crystal and the returning echoes received by another crystal. This system is called *continuous-*

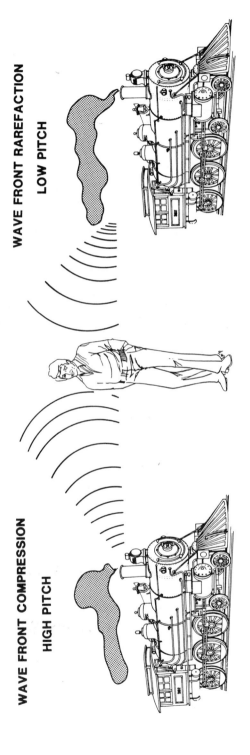

WAVE FRONT RAREFACTION

LOW PITCH

WAVE FRONT COMPRESSION

HIGH PITCH

DOPPLER EFFECT

Figure 1.1 Doppler effect. The whistle of a train coming toward a person will have a higher pitch due to compression of sound waves; the whistle of a train moving away from him will have a lower pitch. If the frequencies of the whistle and the perceived note are known, the speed of the train can be estimated using the doppler formula (see text).

5

wave Doppler echocardiography. In another Doppler system, short pulses of ultrasound with pulse repetition frequencies of 5–10 kHz are used for measurements of blood velocity. This system is called _pulsed Doppler echocardiography._

Doppler echocardiography quantitates and displays visually the frequency shift of the echoes returning from the heart. This procedure can be done by comparing the frequency spectrum of the returning echoes with that of the transmitted ultrasound frequency. The magnitude and direction of the Doppler shift are estimated in a phase detector circuit that compares the returned and transmitted ultrasound frequencies. The Doppler shift signal is passed through a "zero crossing counter" to obtain a time interval histogram (Fig. 1.2). A zero crossing is the instant in time when the Doppler shift signal passes through its zero intensity level. A dot is printed on the strip chart for each zero crossing event so that the location of a particular dot above or below the zero flow velocity baseline is directly proportional to the Doppler shift frequency. The higher the Doppler shift frequency, the farther away the dot will be from the baseline. Dots above the baseline indicate flow toward the transducer, and dots below the baseline indicate flow away from it. Such a dot pattern creates a time interval histogram that can identify blood flow characteristics. A well-streamlined blood flow produces a smooth, uniform Doppler shift, whereas a turbulent flow produces a widely dispersed dot pattern. From the smooth Doppler spectral display, one can estimate the maximum or mean Doppler shift and the velocity of blood flow. The maximum frequency or velocity estimator uses an envelope around the total spectrum for an instantaneous display

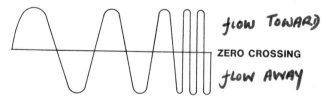

flow TOWARD

ZERO CROSSING

flow AWAY

Figure 1.2   Zero crossing counter. Every time the sound wave passes through the zero intensity a dot is printed. The faster it crosses the zero level, the higher the frequencies registered on the graph.

of peak frequencies or velocities. Many modern Doppler systems use computer-based spectrum analysis. By the use of fast Fourier or discrete Fourier transform, individual frequency components of the Doppler flow signals are separated and plotted. The resultant recording of spectral output gives the directional and quantitated Doppler shift directly related to the blood flow. Doppler equipment also has an audio output that emits sounds in the range of 4–5 kHz, corresponding to the spectrum of Doppler shifts produced by normal or disturbed flow.

The Doppler Formula

Blood flow velocity can be quantitated if the frequency of the transmitted ultrasound beam and the Doppler frequency shift of the returning echo are known. The Doppler equation represents the relationship between frequency shift, maximum velocity, and the angle between the axis of the incident ultrasound beam and the direction of the maximum velocity vectors of the bloodstream that is being measured. The time course of the blood velocity can be calculated from the following equation:

$$V_{max} = \frac{C.\Delta f_{max}}{2.f.\cos\Theta} = \frac{1.54 \times \text{Doppler shift (max)}}{2 \times \text{transducer frequency} \times \cos\Theta}$$

where V_{max} is the instantaneous maximum velocity of the bloodstream (in centimeters per second), C is the velocity of sound in the tissues ($1.54 \cdot 10^5$ cm/sec), f_{max} is the instantaneous maximum frequency shift obtained from the spectrum analyzer (in hertz), f is the frequency of the incident ultrasonic beam (in hertz), and $\cos\Theta$ is the cosine of the angle between the axis of the transmitted ultrasonic beam and the direction of the maximum velocity vectors. From this equation, it is evident that measurement of all instantaneous maximum velocities and consequent total profiling of the velocity pattern of bloodstreams across cardiac valves is best done when the incident ultrasonic beam is directed parallel to the maximal velocity vectors of blood flow, so that $\cos\Theta$ approximates 1 in all calculations. When $\cos\Theta$ is 1, it has been calculated that a Doppler shift of 2.6 kHz indicates the maximum velocity of the blood flow to be 1 m/sec when a Doppler transmitting frequency of 2 MHz is used.

$$\text{Velocity} = \frac{1.54 \times \text{Doppler shift}}{2 \times \text{transducer frequency} \times \cos \Theta}$$

$$= \frac{1.54 \times 2.6}{2 \times 2 \times 1} = 1.001 \text{ m/sec}$$

Many of the new Doppler systems give a fully computed gray-scale spectral display calibrated in meters per second so that the instantaneous velocities can be read directly.

Obstruction of the flow of blood results in an increase in velocity. Pressure increases proximal and decreases distal to the obstruction. This pressure gradient across an obstruction can be quantitatively assessed by Doppler measurement of the velocity of blood flow across the obstruction. The change in flow rate with time across an obstruction can be determined by the Bernoulli equation, which takes into account the convective acceleration and the viscous friction during passage of fluids through a tube. Since the velocity profile across the stenotic valves is flat, the viscous friction may be neglected and a simple modified formula used to measure the gradient.

$$\Delta P = V^2 \times 4$$

where ΔP is the pressure gradient and V is the instantaneous velocity of blood flow. This formula is extensively used in all Doppler echocardiographic calculations. However, it should be pointed out that the pressure gradient may be underestimated when an orifice diameter is reduced to 3.5 mm or less, especially for lower velocities (<3 m/sec). However, most of the hemodynamic calculations in cardiology are for valve orifices with a diameter greater than 3.5 mm.

CONTINUOUS WAVE-DOPPLER ECHOCARDIOGRAPHY

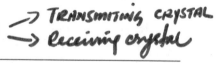
→ TRANSMITTING CRYSTAL
→ receiving crystal

The continuous-wave system uses a continuous stream of ultrasound transmitted from a piezoelectric crystal toward the heart. The ultrasound is back-scattered from the blood cells, and the movements of the latter produce a Doppler shift of ultrasound frequency. The receiving transducer picks up the reflected ultrasound, and the Doppler equipment estimates the direction and extent of Doppler shift. The receiving and transmitting transducers are mounted side by side. The Doppler shift can occur at any depth in the human body during the passage of the echo beam. A maximum shift in the path of the Doppler ultrasound beam may be noted without knowing the depth at which the maximum Doppler shift occurred. This phenomenon is referred to as *range ambiguity*. However, when the anatomic structures through which the echo beam passes are simultaneously imaged using two-dimensional echocardiography, or when the transducer is directed to known anatomic structures, it is generally possible to locate the probable site(s) of the blood flow producing the maximum Doppler shift. An advantage of this technique is its ability to quantitate higher-velocity jets in the heart and great vessels. Continuous-wave Doppler transducers have long been used to measure aortic flow velocity. The incorporation of continuous-wave Doppler capability into the two-dimensional echo system has made it easier to estimate the severity of valvar stenosis, coarctation of the aorta, and instantaneous pressure gradients with considerable accuracy.

PULSED DOPPLER ECHOCARDIOGRAPHY — *SAME CRYSTAL TRANSMIT/RECEIVED*

The pulsed Doppler system uses pulsed ultrasound with a duration of 1 μsec and a frequency of 5–10 kHz. The transducer emits individual pulses. Knowing the velocity of sound through tissues, a depth gating mechanism selectively analyzes the returning signals received during a preselected time. For instance, if the area of interest is at the mitral valve orifice at a depth of 15 cm from the transducer, sound waves traveling at a speed of 1.5 mm/μsec will take 100 μsec to travel from the transducer to the mitral orifice and another 100 μsec to return to the receiver. The "range-gating" mechanism selectively analyzes only the pulses returning 200 μsec after the transmission of each pulse, so that Doppler shifts occur-

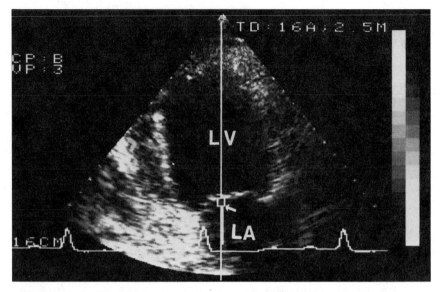

Figure 1.3 Range/depth gating in pulsed Doppler echocardiography. The white line passing through the center of the left ventricle (LV) represents the direction of the Doppler beam. The small box (arrow) seen on the left atrial (LA) side of the mitral valve is the sample volume or range cell. The gating mechanism in the pulsed doppler system receives signals only from this area. The range cell can be moved up and down to detect the flow in various parts of the heart.

ring at the level of the mitral valve orifice alone are detected (Fig. 1.3). In pulsed Doppler echocardiography, the same transducer element transmits and receives the ultrasound: The transmitted pulse should travel to the gated distance and return to be sensed before the next pulse is transmitted. Since only one pulse at a time can traverse the heart, the pulse repetition frequency depends on the depth to which each pulse has to travel. When the sampling is done from deeper locations, the pulse repetition frequency has to be reduced. A signal is usually placed in the Doppler beam indicating the site from which the returning pulses are analyzed. The area sampled is called the *sample volume* or *range cell*, and the technique is called *depth gating*. The depth at which the sample volume is placed can be adjusted by inserting a gate delay interval of 13 μsec/cm of depth. This technique, called *range gating*, enables sampling from various parts of the heart.

For an accurate determination of peak velocities, the pulse repetition frequency or sampling rate has to be at least twice the highest expected Doppler shift frequency, which corresponds to the highest-flow velocity. Hence, at higher depths with low pulse repetition frequency, only low-velocity blood flows can be measured; the high-velocity measurements are erratic. If the pulse repetition frequency is increased so that more than one pulse traverses the heart at the same time, the receiving mode cannot identify the timing of transmission of each pulse, so that the depth to which the pulse has traveled cannot be estimated. This situation produces range ambiguity (or loss of depth information). When the frequency of the Doppler shift (fd) exceeds one-half of the sampling or pulse frequency (fs) the fs is substracted to give a negative fd. The resulting ambiguity, called *aliasing*, causes confusion in clinical applications of pulsed Doppler. To avoid confusion, the back-scattered signal must be sampled before the next pulse is transmitted. Thus, at greater depths, fs must be lower. The maximum radial velocity (v_{max}) at a depth (D) may be expressed as

$$v_m \, D = \frac{c^2}{8f_0}$$

where f_0 is the ultrasonic frequency of the transducer. For an f_0 of 2 MHz in the instrument, one can measure velocities of up to 1.7 m/sec at a depth of 2–8 cm and velocities of 1.1 m/sec at 8–12 cm. Many pulsed Doppler systems can measure blood velocities of up to 1.7 m/sec at 9 cm in depth and up to 1.1 m/sec at 12 cm in depth. This measure corresponds to an fs of 8.6 kHz at depths of less than 9 cm and of 5.7 kHz at depths of more than 9 cm. Pulsed Doppler systems can be used at high pulsing rates (>10 kHz) and still maintain some degree of depth localization. But the velocity profiles obtained show a spurious picture of bidirectional flow called *frequency aliasing*. This picture is analogous to the apparent counterclockwise rotation of the spokes of a wheel on a vehicle moving forward at high speeds in motion pictures. During frequency aliasing (Fig. 1.4), the top part of the velocity recording

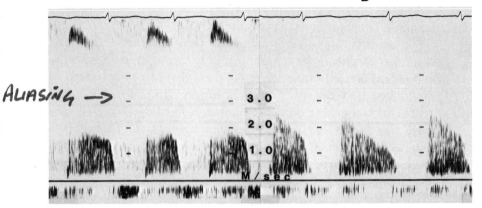

A   B

ALIASING —>

3.0

2.0

1.0

M/sec

Figure 1.4 Panel A shows a Doppler velocity tracing of diastolic mitral flow in a patient with rheumatic mitral stenosis. The use of the pulsed Doppler technique resulted in frequency aliasing. The top of the velocity tracing (>1.7 m/sec) has been snipped off. *Celippri* However, switching over to the continuous-wave Doppler techniques resulted in a recording of peak velocities (panel B).

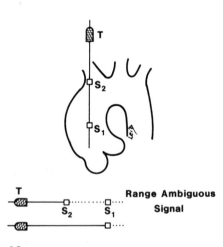

T

S₂

S₁

T   **Range Ambiguous**
S₂   S₁   **Signal**

Figure 1.5 Extended pulsed Doppler technique. In pulsed Doppler echocardiography, the fs has to be at least twice the highest expected Doppler shift frequency. Hence, at higher depths, one can measure only low velocities due to frequency aliasing (see text). However, if another sample volume (S₂) is added, the fs is doubled at the level of the sample volume (S₁) due to range ambiguous signals of S₂. A total of four such sample volumes can be added to multiply the original fs. This procedure enables measurement of velocities up to 5 m/sec at depths of up to 17 cm.

12

is cut off and is turned down to make it look as if there are both positive and negative Doppler shifts. One can even mistake it for a markedly turbulent flow. It is important to know that pulsed Doppler echocardiography at high pulsing rates can produce both range and frequency ambiguities. However, when only positive Doppler shifts are expected, one can mark the negative, ambiguous lower part of the velocity recording on top of the initial Doppler shift recording. Thus, the range of pulsed Doppler velocity recordings can be extended to twice its original limit. In the extended pulsed Doppler technique, gating is done simultaneously in up to four different depths (Fig. 1.5). Pulse repetition frequency can thus be increased stepwise. This system is also known as *high pulse repetition frequency (PRF) Doppler.* The highest Doppler shift occurring at any of the four depths will be recorded as the maximum Doppler shift. This procedure facilitates the measurement of velocities up to 5 m/sec at a depth of 17 cm.

Special types of Doppler equipment are modified to permit sampling from many points on the Doppler beam simultaneously. These are the multigate pulsed Doppler systems. When multiple sample volumes are placed across a large vessel such as the aorta, the flow patterns as well as the diameter of the vessel can be assessed. Some workers have also attempted to color-code the Doppler shift frequencies for easy identification of high-velocity signals.

2

TECHNIQUE
OF DOPPLER ECHO
RECORDING

PROJECTION

A_V — Apical 5 chambers
Suprasternal
Apical Long Axis
Parasternal (OLD PEOPLE) < Lt / Rt

m_V — Apical 4 chambers
Apical Long Axis.

T_V — Apical 4 chambers
Apical Long Axis
Parasternal Short Axis

P_V — PARASTERNAL SHORT AXIS

L → R Chunting — Apical 4 chambers
Subcostal 4 . (child)

SELECTION OF DOPPLER EQUIPMENT

Doppler echocardiography forms part of the two-dimensional echocardiographic examination. For reasons discussed in Chapter 1, Doppler equipment, alone or in combination with M-mode echocardiography, is inadequate for measuring intracardiac flow velocities. An ideal system should provide for real-time visual display of the two-dimensional echo image when the Doppler sample volume is being placed. This capability ensures proper placement of the sample volume in relation to intracardiac structures as well as to heart motion with cardiac and respiratory cycles. An alternative to the real-time display capability is one in which once the sample volume is in the correct position, the image can be frozen and Doppler measurements made. When aliasing is observed, extended pulsed or continuous-wave Doppler echocardiography is required. Measurement of aortic flow velocity, especially in older subjects, may be done from the suprasternal notch or the right parasternal border. Two-dimensional echo images from these approaches are often of poor quality for proper placement of a sample volume. Hence, dual-crystal, continuous-wave Doppler transducers are preferred. These transducers which are quite small, can easily be placed in the suprasternal notch and the intercostal spaces without discomfort to the patient. A two-dimensional echocardiographic system with pulsed Doppler and an extended pulsed or continuous-wave Doppler facility is adequate for most cardiovascular examinations. An additional dual-crystal, continuous-wave Doppler transducer facility broadens the system considerably.

Until recently, simple time interval histograms and maximal and mean velocity estimators alone were used to display Doppler frequency shifts. Such systems are inadequate for correctly judging transducer direction in relation to the maximal velocity vectors of the bloodstream under measurement and for precise measurement of instantaneous velocity. A high-resolution spectrum analyzer with a wide dynamic range and a strip chart recorder with gray-scale capability are a must for all modern Doppler systems. It is advantageous if the output of the spectrum analyzer computes

17

the Doppler shift to the velocity of blood flow and records the latter as meters per second, so that further calculations are not required.

Doppler examinations are done to assess blood flow velocities across the heart valves, the intracardiac defects, or in the great vessels. A comprehensive assessment by clinical and two-dimensional echocardiographic examinations is helpful in planning the Doppler study. Doppler examination is preferably restricted to procedures such as measuring mitral diastolic flow velocity when mitral stenosis is suspected or scanning the anterior border of the interventricular septum in order to rule out a ventricular septal defect.

PATIENT POSITION AND DOPPLER ECHO WINDOWS

A comfortable couch for the patient and a quiet room are essential for the Doppler study. The aim is to measure maximum Doppler shifts at selected locations inside the heart or great vessels. This procedure can be done only if the echo beam is directed parallel to the direction of blood flow. Apex views of the heart, obtained with the patient in the left lateral decubitus position, are commonly obtained for Doppler studies across the mitral and tricuspid valves. The apical four-chamber view, apical five-chamber view (with the aorta in view), and apical long-axis view are most suitable for Doppler flow studies of the mitral valve. Shifting the transducer medially to position it over the right ventricular apex helps to direct the beam toward the tricuspid orifice in the right ventricular inflow view. Some investigators prefer to use the parasternal short-axis view of the heart at the aortic level for studying flow velocity across the tricuspid valve. This view is also suitable for the study of flow patterns across the pulmonary valve and the main pulmonary artery. Upward and medial angulation of the transducer brings the pulmonary valve into view, and further manipulations bring the right ventricular outflow tract, pulmonary valve, and main pulmonary artery near the axial plane. Some investigators

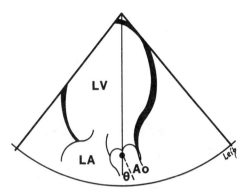

Figure 2.1 The apical long-axis view of the heart is often employed for measurement of flow velocities across the aortic valve. Note that the echo beam and the direction of the central aortic jet are in different directions. When the Doppler shift is used for the calculation of central aortic flow velocity, the cosine θ angle should be measured and used for all calculations. LV, left ventricle; LA, left atrium; Ao, aorta.

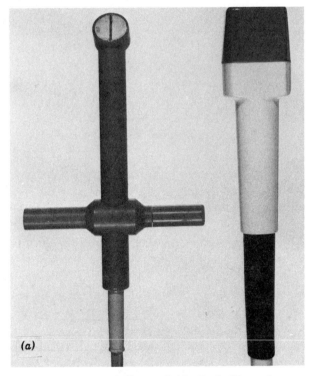

(a)

Figure 2.2 (*a*) A commercially available Pedoff continuous-wave Doppler transducer (left) and a two-dimensional Echo Doppler transducer with capability for simultaneous pulsed or continuous-wave Doppler recordings (right). (*b*) A close up of the two transducers to indicate their dimensions.

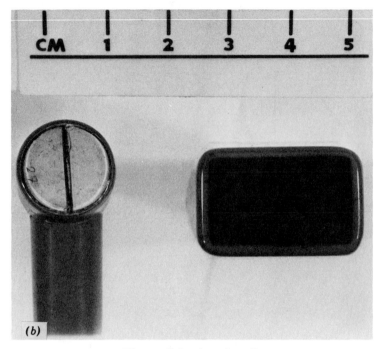

Figure 2.2   (*continued*)

have used this view to examine the flow patterns in patent ductus arteriosus.

Measurement of aortic flow velocities from a precordial approach may be difficult. The apical views in which the Doppler beam can be aligned parallel to the direction of aortic flow are the apical long-axis and the five-chamber views (Fig. 2.1). In older patients, the aorta often takes off at an acute angle, so that the alignment of the Doppler beam from the apex to the direction of blood flow is difficult. The suprasternal window has been used for this purpose. The patient lies on the back with a pillow under the shoulders so that the neck is hyperextended. The transducer is placed in the suprasternal notch to image the ascending aorta where the sample volume is placed. When placement of the two-dimensional echocardiographic Doppler transducer is uncomfortable for the patient, a small dual-crystal, continuous-wave Doppler transducer should be used (Fig. 2.2). This transducer may be easily placed in the suprasternal notch and directed anteriorly caudad and to the right to obtain the ascending aortic flow velocity. Despite the use of this transducer, however, the quality of Doppler signals in an elderly patient with a dilated, tortuous aorta may be poor. We have demonstrated that a right parasternal approach is often ideal for measurement of aortic flow velocity. The patient is made to lie in the right lateral decubitus position. The small continuous-wave transducer is placed in the right second sternal border. Directing it posteriorly, caudad, and to the left will easily align the Doppler beam with the central aortic jet.

In children, the left ventricular and right ventricular outflow tracts may be imaged from the subxiphoid approach, and Doppler studies may be done from this window. Flow patterns across the atrial septal defect can also be measured using this approach.

DOPPLER BEAM PLACEMENT IN CARDIAC IMAGING

The aim of the Doppler study is to measure the maximum Doppler shift at selected locations in the heart, as well as to record the velocity profile of the blood flow. This procedure can be done accurately only if the echo beam is placed within the chamber where the flow velocities are measured and is directed parallel to the direction of blood flow. The angle between the Doppler beam and the true direction of blood flow will determine the accuracy of the velocity measurements. Increasing this angle (cos θ; Fig. 2.1) will result in lower Doppler shifts and underestimation of flow velocity. If the Doppler beam can be aligned to the direction of blood flow or within about 10–20° of angle, and a correct (±5% error) estimate of blood flow velocity can still be made. Increasing this cosine angle decreases the Doppler shift, and at an angle of 60° between the Doppler beam and the direction of blood flow, the velocity measured would be about half the real value. Some systems have facilities for cosine angle correction for calculation of flow velocity, allowing the Doppler beam to be directed conveniently. This capability appears attractive but suffers from the limitation that the angle to be corrected is assessed from a two-dimensional, frozen echo image. Such an image can give the direction of structures in only one tomographic plane, whereas the real angle to be corrected in relation to the direction of flow may be located in an entirely different direction.

Correct alignment of the axis of the incident ultrasonic beam parallel to the maximum velocity vector of blood flow is useful not only in estimating the maximum flow velocity but also in obtaining the velocity profile. For proper assessment of valve narrowing, as well as for calculation of the gradient profile and valve areas, a full-velocity profile of the blood jet should be available. It is important that the specific area where Doppler measurement is made be brought as close to the axial plane of the two-dimensional echo image as possible so that the problem of lateral resolution does not interfere with the Doppler measurement.

DOPPLER RECORDING

When the Doppler beam is properly placed in the two-dimensional echo image, the audio output gives a whistling sound at the time of blood flow and the Doppler display appears on the video screen. If the two-dimensional echo image is frozen at this point, all of the transducer crystals except the one used in the Doppler examination will become inoperative. This situation may improve the quality of Doppler signals. The beam speed of the spectral display is generally kept at 50 mm/sec. The quality of the spectral display may be improved by the following maneuvers:

1. *Baseline adjustment and calibration.* The flow of blood toward the transducer will produce a spectral display above the baseline; flow away from the transducer, below it. Hence, once the spectral display is clearly seen, the baseline should be shifted up or down to bring the display into full view. The calibration of the signal should also be adjusted so that the Doppler pattern is small enough to fill about half of the display width. Peak frequencies may not be adequately recorded if the beam speed is too slow or if the spectral display is too big or too small.

2. *Rejection of low-frequency noises.* Doppler signals may have interfering low-frequency wall motion artifacts and background noise. Wall motion filters are provided in the equipment and can be adjusted to cut down frequencies of 200–600 Hz (Fig. 2.3). Reduction of background noise can be done by careful use of the reject circuit (Fig. 2.4). This circuit should be used sparingly so that the high-frequency components of the spectral display are not attenuated.

3. *Gray-scale compression.* The output of the spectrum analyzer can be best recorded when gray-scale display capability is available. The spectrum analyzer operates in descrete time and frequency. A correct trend shows dense blackening of the apices of the Doppler velocity peaks indicating the highest frequency signals. The amplitude compression of the spectrum analyzer adjusts the gray-scale quality of the display. This quality should be adjusted to obtain a gray-scale display with maximum graying or blackening of the upper margin of each velocity peak (Fig. 2.5).

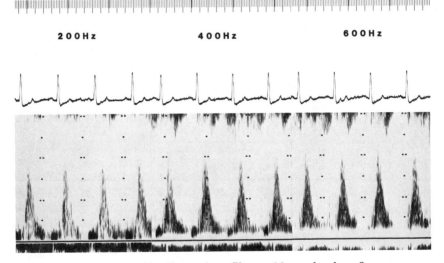

200Hz   **400Hz**   **600Hz**

Figure 2.3 Use of wall motion filters. Note the low-frequency wall motion artifact on either side of the baseline in the first panel. This artifact is reduced by the use of 400- to 600-Hz filters in the second and third panels.

Once the spectral display is properly adjusted and the velocity profile is of high quality, the Doppler beam should be slowly moved across the area under measurement over a 10–20° arc to scan for the highest Doppler shift. The direction of the highest-velocity vector may not often be judged accurately from the two-dimensional echo image alone, especially in the presence of valvar stenosis. The operator should use both the audio output and the spectral display to ascertain that all of the high-frequency components of the Doppler shift are obtained. The output should be recorded on videotape and on a strip chart at speeds of 50 and

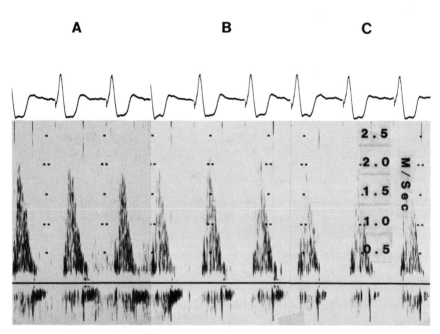

Figure 2.4   Use of the reject mode for attenuation of background noise. This facility should be used sparingly, since it may reject many frequencies in the spectral display, as is evident in panels B and C. Panel A shows adequate rejection of background noise to retain a good spectral display.

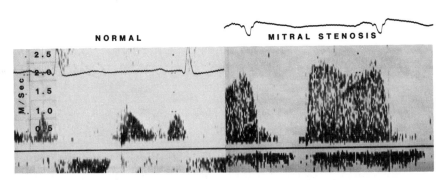

Figure 2.5 Doppler velocity profile of diastolic blood flow through the mitral valve from a normal subject and from a patient with mitral stenosis. Note the blackening of the upper border of both tracings, indicating that the highest Doppler shift frequencies have been recorded in the spectral display. This blackening ensures that the direction of the Doppler beam is parallel to the axis of blood flow.

100 mm/sec, respectively. A simultaneously recorded electrocardiogram is used to time the cardiac events. The echocardiographic window used and the location of the sample volume should be specified in each recording. The audio output should also be recorded on the videotape. With each Doppler recording, a record of the two-dimensional echo image with the Doppler beam direction and the location of the sample volume should also be obtained.

The technique of recording the Doppler velocity spectral display can be summarized in three steps.

Step 1. Align the Doppler beam parallel to the direction of blood flow in the two-dimensional echo image for optimal audio and visual displays.

Step 2. Freeze the two-dimensional echo image and adjust the baseline, calibration factor, wall motion filter, reject mode, and gray-scale compression.

Step 3. (A) Obtain a video recording of the audio and visual displays and the two-dimensional image. (B) Obtain a strip chart recording of the spectral Doppler tracing and the two-dimensional echo image.

RECORDING HIGH-VELOCITY FLOWS — *CW Doppler*

When the blood flow is beyond the range of the pulsed Doppler facility on the spectral display tracing, the top of each velocity trace seems to be trimmed off and the upper part of the display appears at the top of the paper in an inverted manner. This time, if the facility for continuous-wave Doppler exists, the correct velocity measurement may be obtained by switching to it. Otherwise, a high pulsed repetition frequency or an extended pulsed Doppler mode (Fig. 1.5) should be used. The baseline is brought to the bottom of the TV screen, and a second sample is placed in the Doppler beam to double the pulse repetition frequency. If aliasing persists, the number of sample volumes, and consequently the number of pulse repetition frequencies, must be increased. Equipment is now available in which the pulsing frequency can be increased up to five times for measuring higher-velocity jets. This technique has the advantage of locating the site of maximum Doppler shift frequency.

3

DOPPLER EXAMINATION OF MITRAL VALVE FUNCTION

Diagnostic ultrasound was first used for M-mode imaging of the mitral valve and for the diagnosis of mitral stenosis. Subsequently, it was found that the M-mode criteria for quantitation of mitral stenosis are not reliable. The advent of two-dimensional echocardiography provided a means of imaging the mitral valve orifice in the short-axis plane. This view can image the actual cross sections of the narrowed mitral orifice, provided the two-dimensional echocardiographic fan is sectioning the narrowest portion of the orifice. The technique, although often useful, has limitations imposed by the marked structural distortion resulting from heavy calcification and subvalvar disease. In such situations, Doppler measurements of the diastolic mitral gradient provide ancillary means to assess the severity of mitral stenosis.

The echocardiographic diagnosis of mitral regurgitation can only be suspected from indirect evidence such as a dilated, hyperdynamic left ventricle or increased movement of the left atrial walls. In contrast, a Doppler recording obtained from the left atrial side of the mitral valve makes the diagnosis with ease and accuracy. A careful Doppler evaluation is reported to provide a rough quantitation of the severity of mitral regurgitation.

TECHNIQUE

A left ventricular apex view showing either the four-chamber, long-axis or the two-chamber cross section of the heart may be used for two-dimensional imaging of the mitral valve. Once the mitral valve is seen perpendicular to the axial plane, the pulsed Doppler module is switched on. The sample volume is carefully placed so that it is on the ventricular side of the mitral valve funnel during diastole. This position enables one to measure the maximum diastolic flow velocities across the mitral valve. The audio signal of the Doppler machine will produce noise corresponding to the flow pattern and is generally lower-pitched. The spectral display will show a Doppler flow pattern above the zero baseline as the blood flows toward the transducer. Placement of

29

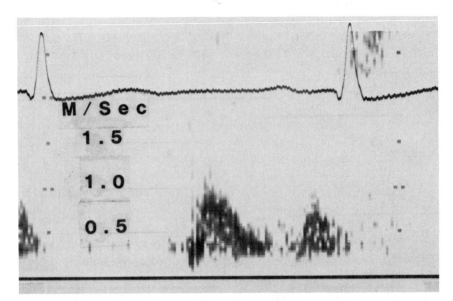

Figure 3.1   Velocity profile of normal blood flow across the mitral valve. Note the high velocity during the rapid inflow phase and atrial systole.

the sample volume too close to the mitral valve will produce loud clicking noises of valve movements, which should be avoided to obtain a good spectral display of diastolic mitral flow. Once the audio output and spectral output signals are found to be acceptable, the two-dimensional echo image may be frozen. The baseline should be shifted to the bottom of the tracing and the calibration adjusted to about 0.5 m/sec. Wall motion filters can be kept at 400 Hz, and the reject mode is carefully used to obtain only the full-velocity profile of the diastolic mitral flow. The normal flow pattern (Fig. 3.1) consists of gradually increasing flow velocity up to 1 m/sec during early diastole during the rapid inflow phase. Subsequently, the velocity falls to about 0.2–0.4 m/sec, to rise again to about 0.6 m/sec during atrial systole. The pattern is similar to the movement of the anterior cusp of the mitral valve in M-mode echocardiographic records. The maximum velocity for normal diastolic flow across the mitral valve varies from 0.6 to 1.3 (mean, 0.9) m/sec.

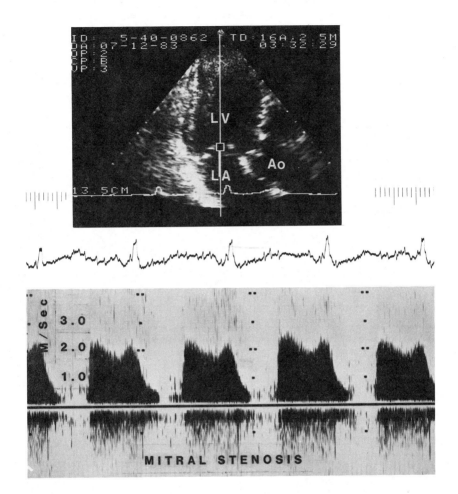

Figure 3.2 Measurement of mitral diastolic flow should be done by imaging the left ventricular apex view of the heart and placing the sample volume on the ventricular side of the mitral funnel (upper panel). The Doppler beam should be placed parallel to the mitral flow. Note that the mitral flow velocity in a patient with mitral stenosis is increased throughout diastole. LA, left artrium; LV, left ventricle; Ao, aorta.

EVALUATION OF MITRAL STENOSIS

Narrowing of the mitral orifice and consequent obstruction to diastolic flow of blood from the left atrium to the left ventricle increase the velocity of blood flow across the mitral valve. Since the effect of obstruction is felt throughout the diastolic period, blood velocity remains high until the end of diastole. When measuring the high-velocity jets of mitral stenosis, the sample volume should be carefully placed just beyond the mitral orifice in the left ventricle (Fig. 3.2). As the diastolic mitral flow velocity rises to more than 1.5 m/sec, the pulsed Doppler tracings will often show frequency aliasing. Extended pulsed Doppler or continuous-wave Doppler will be required to estimate maximal velocity and to obtain a full picture of the diastolic flow pattern across the mitral valve.

Critical mitral stenosis produces peak high velocity jets across the mitral valve measuring more than 2 m/sec (Fig. 3.2). Such

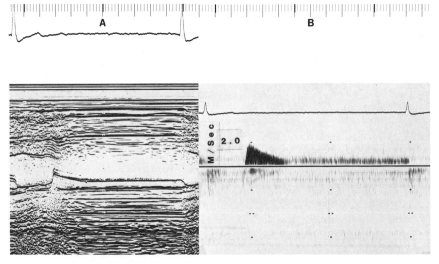

Figure 3.3 Effect of a long cardiac cycle on the mitral flow velocity recording. The velocity comes down to normal levels in spite of mitral stenosis. Note the close resemblance of the velocity tracing to the M-mode tracing of the mitral valve.

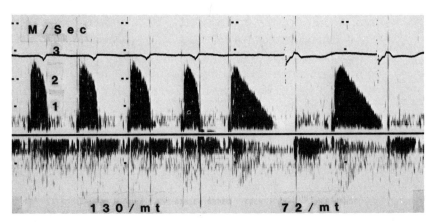

Figure 3.4 Effect of tachycardia on the Doppler velocity profile. Note the high end-diastolic velocity during the heart rate of 110/ min. The end-diastolic velocity came down to normal during a paced heart rate of 72/min. The peak velocities are not substantially different at the two sites.

high-velocity jets can be suspected from the audio signal itself, which gives a higher-pitched noise. The direction of the Doppler beam should be carefully adjusted so that the velocity profile during the entire diastolic period is recorded with good graying of the apices of the spectral display. The diagnostic importance of end-diastolic velocity is considerable, since it reflects the end-diastolic pressure gradient across the mitral valve and correlates with that obtained during cardiac catheterization with simultaneous equisensitive pressures in the left atrium and the left ventricle.

The velocity profile in the presence of critical mitral stenosis shows an early diastolic velocity of more than 2 m/sec. Toward mid-diastole, during the reduced inflow phase, the velocity may decrease slightly, only to rise again during atrial systole. Unlike the normal mitral flow pattern, the velocity remains high at end-diastole, often as high as 2 m/sec. The atrial systolic rise in velocity is not observed if the patient is in atrial fibrillation. The velocity profile in atrial fibrillation resembles the left atrioventricular pressure gradient profile, remaining high during short cardiac cycles and gradually decreasing to near-normal levels in very long cardiac cycles. The pattern closely resembles that of the M-mode echocardiogram of the mitral valve (Fig. 3.3). Tachycardia (Fig. 3.4) and ventricular ectopic beats (Fig. 3.5) may also produce high end-diastolic flow velocity across the mitral valve.

During cardiac catheterization, estimation of the mean diastolic gradient and calculation of the mitral valve orifice area are useful in assessing the severity of mitral stenosis. The mitral velocity data

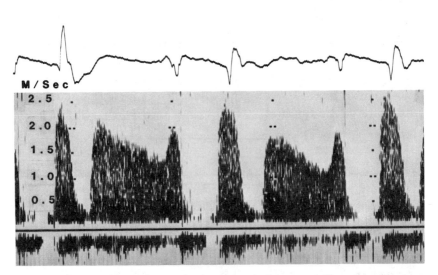

Figure 3.5   Effect of ventricular ectopic beats on diastolic mitral flow velocity. Note the high-velocity recordings during the short diastole following the extra systole.

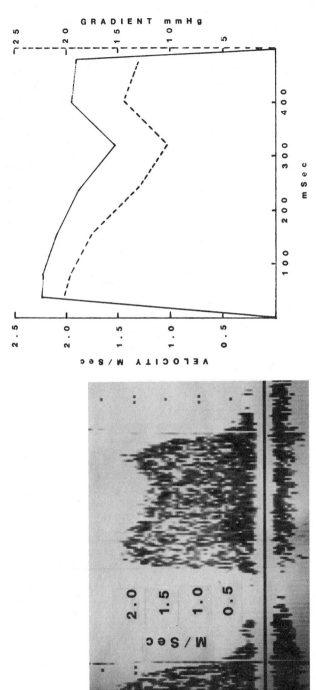

Figure 3.6 Doppler velocity recordings can be used to reconstruct the trend of the transmitted diastolic gradient. In this picture, instantaneous velocity measurements were used at multiple points in diastole to calculate the instantaneous pressure gradients and plot the gradient trend. Note the high end-diastolic gradient.

obtained from Doppler measurements can be used to calculate the instantaneous diastolic gradients across the mitral orifice. Using the formula $\Delta P = V^2 \times 4$ (see "The Doppler Formula" in Chapter 1), end-diastolic mitral velocity can be used to calculate the transmitral end-diastolic gradient (Fig. 3.6). Transmitral gradients calculated from Doppler data have been found to correlate well with the measurements done at the time of cardiac catheterization (Fig. 3.7). In addition to mitral stenosis, a maximum diastolic mitral velocity in excess of 1.5 m/sec may indicate increased flow across the mitral valve, as in anemia, and shunts with augmented transmitral flow, such as ventricular septal defect. However, detailed analysis of the velocity tracings will show that the velocity is high only in early diastole (Fig. 3.8). The velocity rapidly decreases to near zero at end-diastole, indicating the absence of any significant gradient across the mitral valve at end-diastole even at normal heart rates. Availability of full-velocity profile of signals, as well

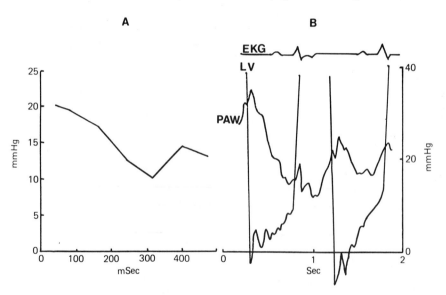

Figure 3.7 Transmitral pressure gradients calculated as shown in Figure 3.6 are compared with the manometric measurements at the time of cardiac catheterization. Note the close correlation between the calculated and measured values. LV, left ventricle; PAW, pulmonary arterial wedge.

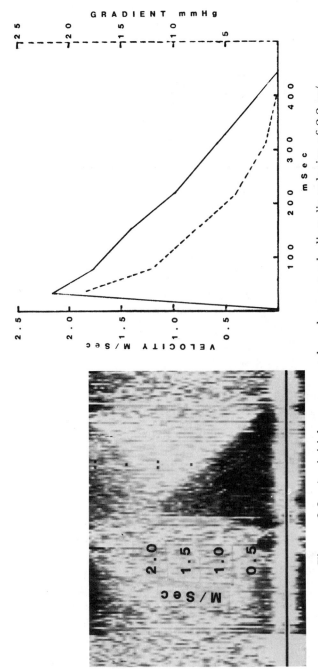

Figure 3.8 An initial assessment based on a peak diastolic velocity of 2.2 m/sec in mitral stenosis was erroneous. A careful analysis of the Doppler data shows that the high initial velocity rapidly decreased to normal. The calculated mitral valve area was 2.1 cm². There was no significant obstruction across the mitral valve on cardiac catheterization. The initial high velocity was found to be due to high cardiac output secondary to anemia.

as the estimation of atrioventricular pressure half-time, will aid in avoiding false-positive diagnoses.

ATRIOVENTRICULAR PRESSURE HALF-TIME

The absence of an early diastolic decrease in mitral velocity is a good index of the severity of mitral obstruction. Hatle and co-workers (1979) demonstrated that the mitral velocity trend during early diastole shows a pattern similar to the mitral valve gradient trend in mitral stenosis, as observed by Libanoff and Rodbard (1966, 1968). The time taken by the atrioventricular pressure gradient to decrease to half of its initial level is termed the *atrioventricular pressure half-time* and provides a good index of the severity of mitral stenosis. This assessment is more accurate than evaluations from the observation of the end-diastolic mitral velocity or end-diastolic pressure gradient, since the atrioventricular pressure half-time is not influenced by changes in cycle length (Fig. 3.3). Since each instantaneous maximum velocity measurement represents the instantaneous transmitral gradient, the spectral display of the velocity profile is used to calculate the atrioventricular pressure half-time. The decrease in the transmitral gradient is exponential, and hence the instantaneous gradients plotted on semilogarithmic graph paper give the time taken by the transmitral gradient to decrease to half of its initial value (Fig. 3.9). Hatle and Angelsen (1982) showed that since the relationship between velocity and pressure is quadratic, the pressure half-time may be calculated by dividing the initial peak velocity by $\sqrt{2}$ ($= 1.41$) and measuring the time taken for the peak velocity to decrease to the latter level.

Libanoff and Rodbard (1966, 1968) found that atrioventricular pressure half-time measured by cardiac catheterization and manometric studies was a reliable and sensitive measure of mitral valve obstruction. Varying heart rates (Fig. 3.10), cardiac output, or the presence of associated mitral regurgitation do not alter this measurement. Hatle and colleagues found that the atrioventricular pressure half-times calculated from Doppler velocity tracings are

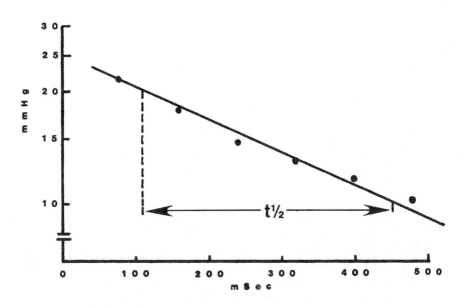

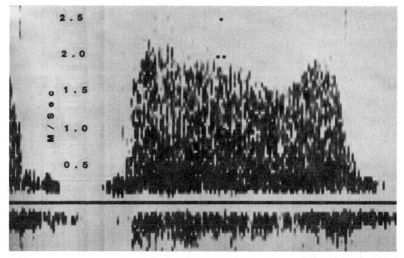

Figure 3.9 Instantaneous velocities from six points in the early part of diastole were used to calculate the instantaneous transmitral gradient. These values were plotted on semilogarithmic paper. Atrioventricular pressure half-time was measured as the time taken for the gradient to decrease by half.

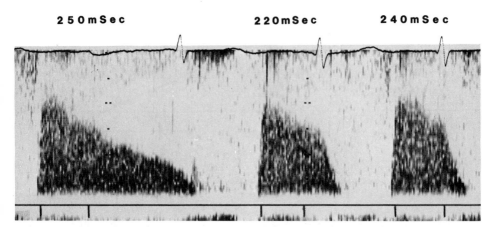

PRESSURE HALF-TIME

Figure 3.10   Doppler velocity recording from a patient with mitral stenosis and atrial fibrillation. Three cardiac cycles with different R-R intervals are shown. Note the different end-diastolic velocities. However, the atrioventricular pressure half-time calculated from each remains similar.

just as reliable as those observed by Libanoff and Rodbard. In normal subjects the half-time varied from 20 to 60 msec, whereas in patients with mitral stenosis it varied from 100 to 400 msec. Pressure half-time varied from 174 to 280 msec in patients with moderate mitral stenosis, but was less than 180 msec in patients with mild stenosis.

MITRAL VALVE AREA DERIVED FROM DOPPLER VELOCITY MEASUREMENTS

The modified Gorlin formula was used to calculate the mitral valve area (MVA) using the mitral valve gradient calculated from the Doppler velocity recordings and the mitral flow rate measured at the time of cardiac catheterization by Holen and colleagues (1977). The data correlated well with those calculated from the hemodynamic data. Later, Hatle and Angelsen (1982) showed that with a pressure half-time of more than 220 m/sec, the valve area was less than 1 cm^2. Hence, we advocate the use of the formula

$$\text{MVA (cm}^2) = \frac{220}{\text{pressure half-time (msec)}}$$

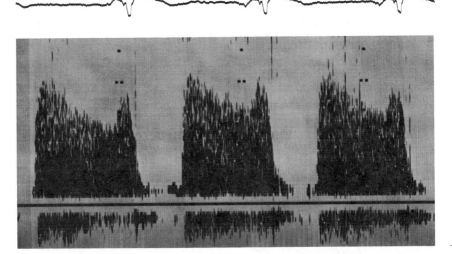

$$\text{MVA}: \frac{220}{t\frac{1}{2}} : \frac{220}{310} : 0 \cdot 7 \text{cm}^2$$

Figure 3.11   Calculation of MVA from Doppler velocity data. Atrioventricular pressure half-time ($t_{1/2}$) may be estimated by plotting the instantaneous pressure gradients (calculated from Doppler measurements). Dividing 220 by $t_{1/2}$ gives the mitral valve area.

for calculation of the mitral valve area from the Doppler velocity measurements alone (Fig. 3.11). The methods described above appear to be quite reliable for assessing the severity of mitral stenosis. However, it should be stressed that the linear relationship between mitral valve area and pressure half-time exists only when the mitral orifice is significantly narrowed.

4

MITRAL REGURGITATION

TECHNIQUE

Mitral regurgitation is a common condition in which the Doppler echo method may be used to identify and quantitate the lesion. The mitral valve and the left atrium are easily brought into the axial plane of the two-dimensional echo image from the apical views. The pulsed Doppler sample volume should be kept on the left atrial side of the mitral valve for detection of the regurgitant jet (Fig. 4.1). In many patients, especially those with cardiomegaly, the mitral valve may be more than 7 cm from the left ventricular apex. Hence, frequency aliasing is commonly observed when the pulsed Doppler technique is used. When the mitral valve is situated beyond 12 cm from the left ventricular apex, the sample volume cannot be placed on the left atrial side of the mitral valve, since the region is beyond the reach of the conventional pulsed Doppler depth gating technique. The extended Doppler facility may overcome this limitation. The detection of mitral regurgitation may also be aided by placing the transducer closer to the left sternal border so that the mitral valve is imaged closer to the transducer. However, this position is not suitable for quantitation of mitral regurgitation velocity, since the echo beam will have a wide angle with the regurgitant jet. When the mitral valve is brought perpendicular to the axial plane of the video screen as seen from the apical views, continuous-wave Doppler may be used for the detection and quantitation of mitral regurgitation, since the beam would not be expected to cross any other bloodstream with the high velocity observed in mitral regurgitation.

The regurgitant jet produces a high-pitched systolic audio signal that is often pansystolic. The spectral display will show a high-velocity jet going away from the transducer (Fig. 4.1). Once the regurgitant jet is identified, it may be necessary to readjust the transducer angle so that the Doppler beam is made parallel to it. Finer adjustments of the transducer can be attempted after freezing the two-dimensional echo image. At this point, the baseline of the spectral display may have to be shifted to the top of the screen. Mitral regurgitant jets nearly always have high velocities. Since they are generally beyond the range of pulsed Doppler capability, the extended pulsed Doppler or the continuous-wave

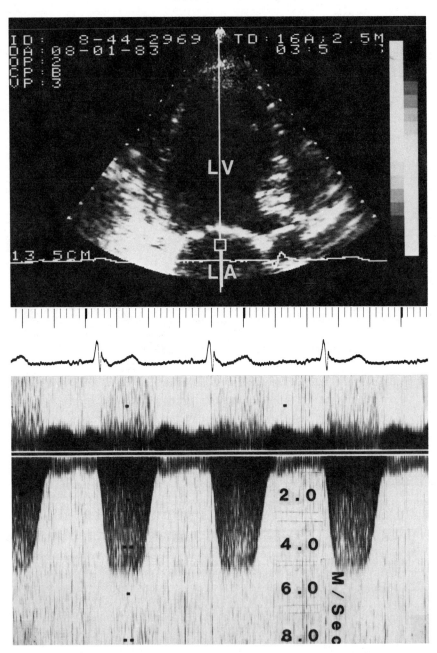

Figure 4.1 Doppler evaluation of mitral regurgitation. The sample volume is placed on the left atrial side of the mitral valve while

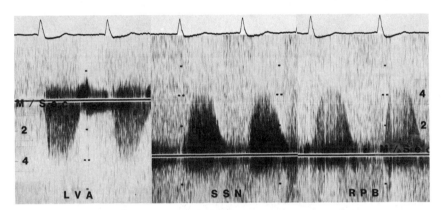

Figure 4.2   Doppler signals from a mitral regurgitation jet recorded from the left ventricular apex (LVA), suprasternal notch (SSN), and right parasternal border (RPB) in a patient with flail posterior cusp. Note the close similarity of the Doppler signal to that seen in aortic stenosis.

Doppler technique should be used. The calibration of the spectral display may also need to be changed to 1 or 2 m/sec/cm. Care should be taken to obtain the full profile of the regurgitant jet, with maximum graying of the peaks of the spectral display. The mitral regurgitant velocities are often in the range of 4–6 m/sec. When the Doppler beam is closer to the interatrial septum, especially while using the continuous-wave Doppler technique, forward flow into the ascending aorta may be detected and an erroneous diagnosis of mitral regurgitation could be made.

←

the Doppler beam is directed perpendicular to it (upper panel). The spectral display of mitral regurgitation obtained with the continuous-wave Doppler technique appears below the baseline (lower panel) and has a peak velocity above 4 m/sec. LV, left ventricle; LA, left atrium.

Similarly, mitral regurgitation due to disease of the posterior mitral cusp may produce a jet directed toward the interatrial system and the aortic root. Velocity profiles similar to those of aortic stenosis may be recorded from the left ventricular apex, suprasternal notch, and right parasternal border (Fig. 4.2). However, detailed analysis of the spectral display (Fig. 4.3) will help one to distinguish the mitral regurgitant jet. Mitral regurgitation commonly starts during the isovolumic contraction period of systole within 40–50 msec after the Q wave of the electrocardiogram, whereas the aortic flow starts only after the aortic valve opens, generally about 80–100 msec after the Q wave. Moreover,

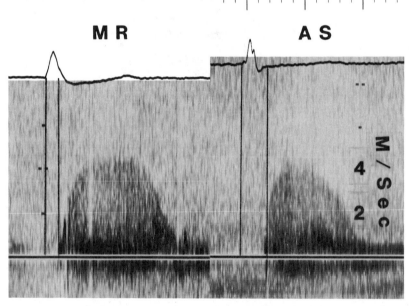

Figure 4.3 Doppler velocity-spectral display of mitral regurgitation (MR) and aortic stenosis (AS). Note its early onset in mitral regurgitation. The regurgitant jet velocity rapidly reaches its maximum and remains there throughout systole. Aortic flow starts later in systole and slowly reaches a peak. Both of the recordings were done from the second right parasternal border using a Pedof dual-crystal, continuous-wave Doppler transducer.

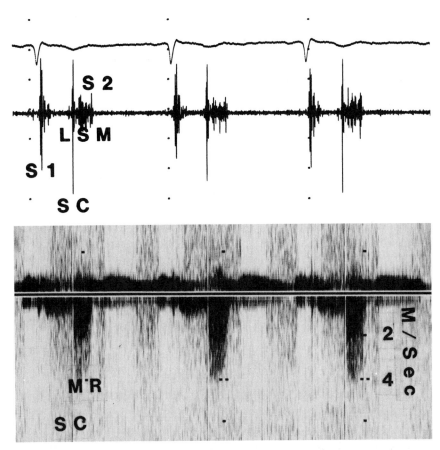

Figure 4.4 Doppler and phono cardiographic recordings from a patient with mitral valve prolapse and late systolic mitral regurgitation (LSM). Note the systolic click (SC) in the phonocardiogram and the corresponding noise signal in the Doppler recording. The mitral regurgitation (MR) recorded by the phonocardiogram and Doppler enchocardiogram corresponds very well in timing.

the spectral display of the mitral regurgitant jet reaches its peak within 40 msec and will often maintain a plateau throughout ventricular systole. Even in patients with mitral valve prolapse or papillary muscle dysfunction, in which mitral regurgitation is not pansystolic, the shape of the spectral display (Fig. 4.4) is generally different from the aortic velocity profile. It should also be kept in mind that high-velocity jets across the aortic valve (>2 m/sec) occur only in left ventricular outflow obstruction and a velocity of more than 4 m/sec indicates a high gradient, whereas mitral regurgitation jets often have a velocity of more than 4 m/sec.

Many workers have used pulsed Doppler mapping of the left atrium for the quantitation of mitral regurgitation. A common technique is to use the pulsed Doppler sample volume. Once the mitral regurgitant jet is detected, the sample volume is gradually shifted more cephalad into the left atrium to determine how far into the left atrial cavity the mitral regurgitant jet is detected. Only in severe mitral regurgitation can it be sensed from the middle of the left atrium. Similarly, placement of the sample volume may be varied from side to side; it can be placed closer to the interatrial septum, in the mid-left atrium, and then in the lateral wall to study the width of the regurgitant jet. The latter technique is of limited use, since the mitral regurgitation jet may often be detected in only one direction. Regurgitation through a small orifice produces a very high-velocity jet. Such regurgitant jets are so small that a full velocity profile may be difficult to obtain. We have found that mitral regurgitation jets with a velocity of more than 5 m/sec often indicate mild mitral regurgitation.

ESTIMATIONS OF LEFT ATRIAL PRESSURES

Hemodynamically, mitral regurgitation occurs from the left ventricle with a high systolic pressure across the regurgitant orifice into the left atrium with lower pressure. One can calculate the pressure difference between the left ventricle (LV) and the left

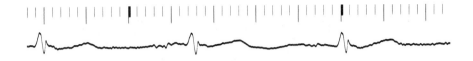

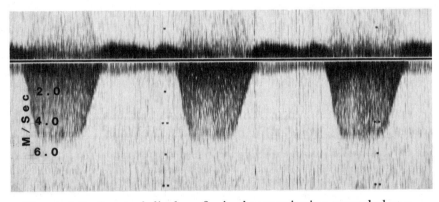

Figure 4.5 Spectral display of mitral regurgitation recorded at a paper speed of 100 mm/sec. Note that the regurgitation starts 40 msec after the beginning of the QRS cycle. It immediately rises to its maximal velocity and remains there until the end of systole. The pattern is different from that of the spectral display of aortic stenosis. The mitral regurgitation velocity of 5 m/sec in this patient was used to calculate the height of the left artrial V wave. Systemic blood pressure was 124/86 mm Hg. The LV-LA gradient was calculated using the formula $\triangle P = V^2 \in 4$, i.e., $5^2 \times 4 = 100$ mg Hg; the LA − V wave is $124 - 100 = 24$ mm Hg. (The height of the left atrial V wave during cardiac catheterization was recorded as 26 mm Hg.)

atrium (LA) using the formula $P = V^2 \times 4$ if the velocity of the regurgitant jet is known. Since the systolic pressure in the left ventricle is same as the arterial pressure in the absence of left ventricular outflow obstruction, it can be estimated using a sphygmomanometer. Once the left ventricular systolic pressure and the LV-LA systolic gradient are known, the left atrial pressure during ventricular systole at the peak of mitral regurgitation can be calculated as the difference between the brachial systolic blood pressure and the estimated LV-LA systolic gradient (Fig. 4.5). This will approximate height of the left atrial V wave. When the left atrial size is normal or only slightly enlarged, the height of the V wave may provide an indication of the severity of mitral regurgitation. However, it is well known that systolic pressure in a large, compliant left atrium may be normal despite severe mitral regurgitation. When mitral stenosis and regurgitation coexist, the velocity recording of the diastolic mitral stenotic jet and the systolic mitral regurgitant jet should be done separately, since the direction of the maximum velocity vectors of these two jets may be different. There may be no problem when extended pulsed Doppler is used, since the sample volume is kept at entirely different locations for these two lesions. However, when continuous-wave Doppler measurements are used, the spectral display of the mitral stenotic and regurgitant jets may appear in the same tracing. However, careful adjustments of the transducer direction will help obtain the accurate velocity profile of each lesion individually.

5

DOPPLER EXAMINATION OF AORTIC VALVE FUNCTION

TECHNIQUE

The velocity profile obtained by Doppler echocardiography in the ascending aorta and in the left ventricular outflow space is useful in diagnosing left ventricular outflow obstruction or aortic regurgitation. The left ventricular outflow tract and the ascending aorta may be easily imaged in children and many adults from the left ventricular apex and the subxyphoid region. The ascending aorta may also be visualized from the suprasternal approach. When the two-dimensional echo image is of good technical quality, the pulsed Doppler sample volume can be placed in the subaortic and supraaortic regions to measure the forward blood flow velocity or to detect retrograde flow in aortic valvular regurgitation. The aortic flow velocity and the cross-sectional area of the aorta are also commonly employed for calculating the cardiac output (see Chapter 10).

In older patients, especially those with emphysema, it is often difficult to direct the Doppler beam parallel to the central aortic jet while imaging from the cardiac apex. The problem may be due to dilatation, unfolding, and tortuosity of the aorta, which may arise at an acute angle from the left ventricle. In this age group, suprasternal imaging of the aorta is also difficult. Under such circumstances, it is preferable to use the small dual-crystal, continuous-wave Doppler transducer from the suprasternal notch or the upper right sternal border. A pillow is placed under the shoulders, and the patient is made to lie on the back, with the head extended and the chin turned to the right side. The transducer is placed in the suprasternal notch and directed caudally, anteriorly, and to the right to align the Doppler beam parallel to the ascending aortic bloodstream (Fig. 5.1). In all older patients, the right sternal border approach should be tried. Here the patient is asked to lie on the right side, and the transducer is placed in the first or second right sternal border. The Doppler beam is directed to the left, posteriorly, and caudally. In older patients, aortic flow velocity is thus best recorded from either the suprasternal notch or the right sternal border.

When the continuous-wave Doppler technique is used to quan-

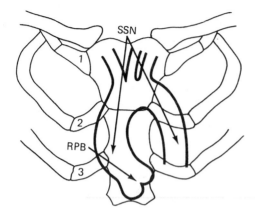

Figure 5.1 Direction of the Doppler beam when the continuous-wave Doppler transducer is kept in the suprasternal notch (SSN) or the right parasternal border (RPB) for measurement of aortic flow velocity. Note that the leftward tilt of the suprasternal transducer detects the descending aortic flow.

titate a valvar lesion, it is important to obtain a high-quality spectral display. The alignment of the Doppler beam with the central aortic jet can be judged from the high-pitched whistling sound of the audio output. Once this sound is clearly heard without any background noise, the baseline is shifted to the bottom of the tracing. The Doppler display will appear above the baseline (Fig. 5.2), since the systolic blood flow is toward the transducer, which is placed in the suprasternal notch or the right sternal border.

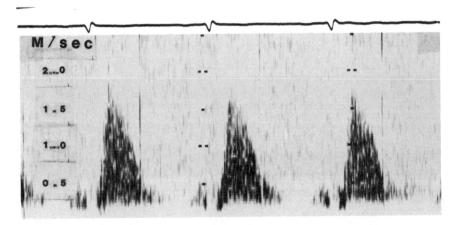

Figure 5.2 Normal aortic flow velocity recording from the right parasternal border. The spectral display shows darkening of the peaks, indicating that the highest frequencies were recorded. The velocity profile rapidly rises to a peak in early systole.

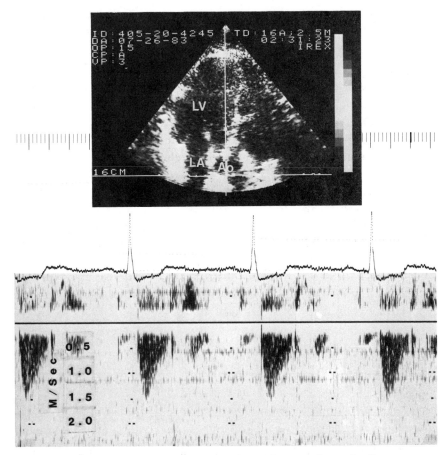

Figure 5.3 Doppler velocity tracing of central aortic flow recorded from the left ventricular apex. The directions of the Doppler beam and the central aortic jet are often not parallel. The Doppler beam is directed toward the left ventricular outflow and the ascending aorta (upper panel). The spectral display (lower panel) appears below the baseline as the flow is directed away from the transducer. Note the early systolic peaking of the normal velocity profile. LV, left ventricle; LA, left atrium; Ao, aorta.

From a more leftward and posterior angulation of the transducer in the suprasternal notch, one may detect a descending aortic blood flow. Here the display of flow directed away from the transducer appears below the baseline. Intermediate positions of the transducer can give a spectral display on both sides of the baseline due to blood flow perpendicular to the Doppler beam in the aortic arch. The Doppler aortic spectral display for systolic flow will appear below the baseline when recorded from the left ventricular apex or the subxiphoid region (Fig. 5.3).

The normal aortic Doppler velocity tracing starts about 100 msec after the Q wave of the electrocardiogram. It rises early to a peak and returns to the baseline toward the end of systole. The highest velocity recorded from any of the three approaches is taken as the true central aortic blood flow velocity. Normal values range from 1.0 to 1.9 ($\overline{m}$ 1.3 ± 0.3) m/sec. They increase in patients with aortic outflow obstruction, as well as in high cardiac output states such as anemia and pregnancy, or with increased stroke volume in aortic regurgitation.

AORTIC STENOSIS

The difficulties encountered in assessing the severity of aortic stenosis by clinical and echocardiographic criteria are well known. In children, the severity of aortic stenosis is often underestimated. Rheumatic aortic stenosis, when present with mitral stenosis, can be missed or its severity underestimated. In older patients, aortic valve sclerosis and calcification may not be easily differentiated from valve stenosis. Impaired left ventricular function due to other causes may reduce the opening movement of a thickened or mildly calcified valve, as observed by two-dimensional echocardiography, resulting in erroneous diagnosis or overestimation of aortic stenosis. In many such instances, estimation of Doppler aortic velocity is of great help in accurate quantitation of aortic valve stenosis.

Narrowing of the aortic valve with obstruction to blood flow from the left ventricle to the ascending aorta results in a high-velocity bloodstream across the aortic valve. The maximal velocity vector is generally best estimated from the ascending aorta. In infants and children, this measurement may be easily done using the left ventricular apex views (apical long-axis or five-chamber view) or subcostal views, or by suprasternal imaging of the ascending aorta. From all three approaches, a good image of the ascending aorta is possible. When the ascending aorta is visualized clearly, it is easy to place the Doppler beam parallel to the central aortic jet. Once the supravalvar region of the ascending aorta is brought near the axial plane of the video screen, the pulsed Doppler sample volume can be placed above the aortic valve. Aortic stenosis will be immediately evident on the spectral display, since the high-velocity jets produce frequency aliasing. The two-dimensional echo image should be frozen and an extended pulsed Doppler or continuous-wave Doppler facility used to measure the maximum velocity of the central aortic bloodstream.

In elderly patients, imaging of the ascending aorta from the left ventricular apex, subxiphoid region, or suprasternal notch is technically difficult. The images, when obtained, are of poor quality. In addition, the depth at which the sample volume has to be placed makes the pulsed Doppler technique of limited value. A small continuous-wave Doppler transducer provides reliable tracings when used from the suprasternal notch or the right parasternal border. In patients with poststenotic dilatation of the aorta, the right sternal border approach generally gives the best results. Aortic stenosis can be suspected by the high-pitched note of the audio output. The sound often has a soft, whistling quality. In severe aortic stenosis, the pitch can be so high as to render the sound almost inaudible. When the audio and spectral displays are satisfactory, the calibration is readjusted to include peak signals. Careful adjustment of the transducer angle will produce a spectral display with the highest frequencies located at the peak of the tracings (Fig. 5.4). Recordings should be done at 50 mm/sec and 100 mm/sec paper speeds, with minimum gray-scale compression.

The aortic blood flow velocity in aortic stenosis is directly related to the pressure gradient resulting from aortic valve narrowing. The maximum systolic gradient from the left ventricle to the aorta can be calculated using the formula $\Delta P = V^2 \times 4$ (see Chapter

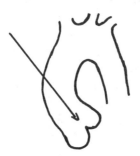

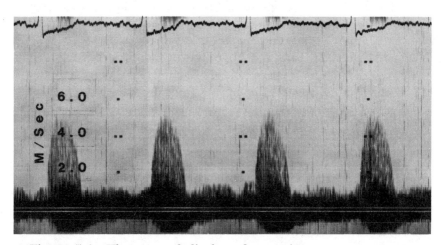

Figure 5.4 The spectral display of a continuous-wave Doppler flow velocity profile in the ascending aorta obtained from the right parasternal border shows a peak velocity of 5 m/sec in a patient with severe aortic stenosis. The estimated gradient of 100 mg Hg compares favorably with the measured peak gradient of 90 mm Hg in this patient.

mp 6

1) and the severity of the aortic stenosis assessed. The correlation between the maximum pressure gradient measured at cardiac catheterization and that estimated from the continuous-wave Doppler velocity signal is excellent. The gradient may be underestimated when the true peak velocity is not obtained. However, experience in our laboratory suggests that the peak velocity is successfully measured if the suprasternal and right parasternal as well as the apical approaches are employed. We have noted that the gradient may be apparently overestimated in comparing the Doppler estimated maximum gradient to the peak-to-peak gradient on a pullback pressure recording from the left ventricle to the aorta. The peak-to-peak gradient is often substantially lower than the instantaneous maximum gradient, with which the Doppler peak velocity is better correlated. The maximum instantaneous gradient across the aortic valve is seldom reported in the routine cardiac catheterization data analysis. The maximum gradient occurs during the early part of systole, when the left ventricular pressure rises briskly and the aortic pressure rise lags behind. It is this maximum instantaneous gradient in early systole that is reflected as the maximum or peak systolic velocity in the Doppler tracings. Mean systolic gradients calculated from Doppler measurements as an average of multiple instantaneous gradients every 40–50 msec and those planimetered from pressure tracings also correlate well. The peak-to-peak systolic gradients are not truly instantaneous, and are generally lower than the maximum systolic gradient because the left ventricular pressure peak reaches a plateau earlier than the aortic pressure (Fig. 5.5). With increasing severity of aortic stenosis, left ventricular peak systolic pressure will be sustained for a longer period, and hence the difference between the maximum systolic and peak-to-peak systolic gradients becomes less. However, it should be stressed that for accuracy the systolic gradient calculated from Doppler velocity measurements should be compared with the maximum systolic gradients in patients with aortic stenosis.

Another potential error in overestimation of the gradient may occur if the velocity profile of mitral regurgitation is mistaken for the aortic flow velocity. This mistake may be avoided with close attention to the time of onset, peak, and shape of the velocity profile. Clinicians and phonocardiographers have stressed that the late peaking of the aortic systolic murmur indicates severe aortic stenosis. Similarly, Hatle and co-workers (1980) showed that increasing severity of aortic stenosis will result in delayed peaking of Doppler aortic velocity tracings (Fig. 5.6). However, the time of the peak velocity in displays does not correspond precisely to the time of the maximal gradient across the aortic valve. The peak flow velocity is out of phase with the peak development of pressure. Murgo and co-workers (1980) have shown that the aortic velocity peaks occur approximately 60 msec after the maximum aortic pressure rises. This delay in velocity peaks is thought to be due

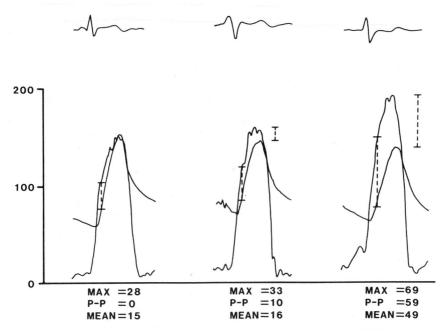

Figure 5.5 Simultaneous left ventricular pressure pulses in three representative patients demonstrate a difference between the maximum (max) and peak-to-peak (P-P) pressure gradients. A considerable discrepancy between them may exist. The peak velocity correlates better with the maximum than with the peak-to-peak gradient, which is more often reported in cardiac catheterization studies.

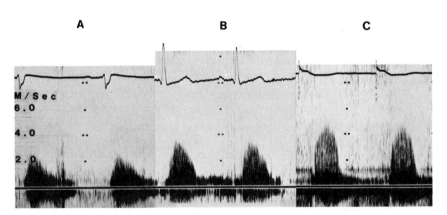

Figure 5.6 Panels A, B, and C show Doppler aortic velocity tracings from three patients with mild, moderate, and severe aortic stenosis respectively. Peak velocities were 2.75, 3.5, and 4.75 m/sec, respectively. The calculated left ventricle-aortic gradients were 30, 49, and 90 mm Hg, and the measured maximum gradients at the time of cardiac catheterization were 36, 50, and 100 mm Hg, respectively. Note the early peaking of the velocity tracing in panel A and the late peaking in panel C (160 and 280 m/sec, respectively, after the beginning of the Q wave on the electrocardiogram). Note the change in shape from a cone (normal) to a truncated cone on the aortic velocity tracing in severe aortic stenosis.

to inertia in the flow velocity. A central aortic flow velocity of more than 2 m/sec indicates left ventricular outflow obstruction. However, one should remember that increased blood flow through a normal aortic valve, as in anemia, can increase aortic flow velocity. Severe aortic stenosis not only produces a peak velocity of more than 4 m/sec but also changes the shape of the spectral display. The normal aortic velocity rises to a peak, immediately comes down to normal, and has a conical shape. In severe aortic stenosis, the apex of the velocity tracing becomes wider and the display has the shape of a truncated cone.

Left ventricular outflow obstruction due to hypertrophic cardiomyopathy, discrete subvalvar stenosis, or supravalvar stenosis can be identified by careful use of the pulsed Doppler sample volume. The area where the aortic velocity increases can be mapped by placing the sample volume at various points in the left ventricular outflow, starting from the left ventricular cavity. Information gathered from the clinical and two-dimensional echocardiographic studies are helpful in planning a careful Doppler examination of the left ventricular outflow tract.

6

AORTIC REGURGITATION

Aortic regurgitation is often an easy clinical diagnosis based on the presence of a characteristic murmur. However, its differentiation from pulmonary regurgitation may prove to be difficult. It is well recognized that no detectable murmur may be present with mild and occasionally even moderate aortic regurgitation. The physical signs in acute aortic regurgitation are also often atypical. The echocardiographic signs of diastolic flutter of the mitral valve or the interventricular septum and the signs of diastolic overload in the left ventricle are useful diagnostic signs. Since the advent of Doppler echocardiography, many workers have attempted to quantitate aortic regurgitation by plotting the Doppler velocity profile of systolic and diastolic flow patterns in the descending aorta. A continuous-wave Doppler transducer kept in the suprasternal notch has been used to measure the velocity profile of the descending aortic flow. It was reported that in aortic regurgitation, an exaggerated reverse flow pattern was observed in the descending aorta. The area under the systolic and diastolic velocity tracings was planimetered, since it represents the distance a column of blood moves forward and backward. The ratio of the forward and backward movements of the descending aortic blood flow correlated well with the severity of aortic regurgitation estimated by supravalvar aortography. However, such estimations are of limited value in the presence of aortic stenosis and cannot differentiate other causes of aortic runoff, such as patent ductus arteriosus.

The introduction of pulsed Doppler echocardiography has made precise identification of aortic regurgitation possible by the placement of the sample volume beneath the aortic valve (Fig. 6.1). The patient lies in the left lateral decubitus position, and a left ventricular apical long-axis view is imaged on the video screen. In this view, the Doppler beam can be placed parallel to the direction of the aortic regurgitant jet. The sample volume is kept under the aortic valve, and the pulsed Doppler technique is used to detect the regurgitant jet. An aortic regurgitant jet produces a high-pitched, hissing noise that may be detected if one listens carefully. In its milder form, the jet can be localized so that small changes in Doppler beam direction, such as with normal respirations, could make it appear on the display screen only intermittently. Since the velocity of the aortic regurgitant jet is high, an adaptive or

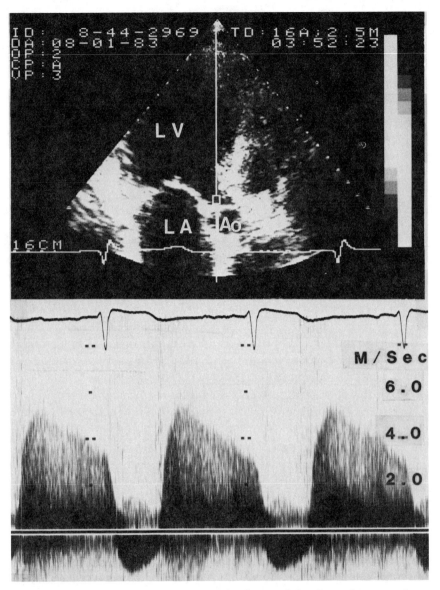

Figure 6.1 Aortic regurgitation is detected by Doppler examination of the subaortic region using the pulsed Doppler technique. The sample volume is placed beneath the aortic valve to sense the diastolic regurgitant jet (upper panel). However, the quantitation of maximal velocities and full profiling of the regurgitation (lower panel) can be obtained only by the continuous-wave Doppler

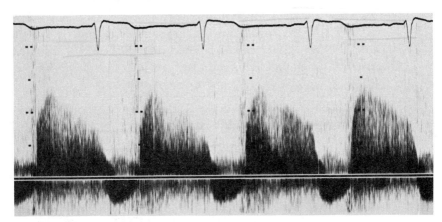

Figure 6.2 It is useful to calculate the left ventricular end-diastolic pressure form the end-diastolic velocity of the aortic regurgitation jet. The end-diastolic aortic-left ventricular gradient is calculated from the end-diastolic velocity using the formula $\Delta P = V^2 \times 4$. When this value is subtracted from the systemic diastolic blood pressure as determined by a sphygmomanometer, one can obtain the estimated left ventricular end-diastolic pressure. However, care should be taken to select Doppler traces with good spectral displays for this purpose. The first two cardiac cycles show an absence of blackening of the upper border of the trace, and the end-diastsolic velocity appears to be spuriously low. However, the last complex shows a correct gray-scale display with a high end-diastolic velocity.

←

technique, as shown in this example. The extended pulsed Doppler technique may also be used. Calculating the end-diastolic aorta-left ventricular gradient and subtracting it from the brachial diastolic blood pressure gives the left ventricular end-diastolic pressure. LV, left ventricle; LA, left atrium; Ao, aorta.

continuous-wave Doppler technique is required to obtain its true velocity profile. Only spectral displays with distinct blackening of the upper border should be used for quantitative measurements.

The jet of aortic regurgitation produces a box-shaped velocity spectral display (Fig. 6.1). It is maximum in early diastole and gradually decreases. Early diastolic velocity varies from 4.0 to 5.5 m/sec. A good-quality spectral display can be used to calculate the aortic to left ventricular diastolic gradient at various times in diastole. Subtracting the calculated end-diastolic gradient from the measured diastolic arterial blood pressure gives the left ventricular

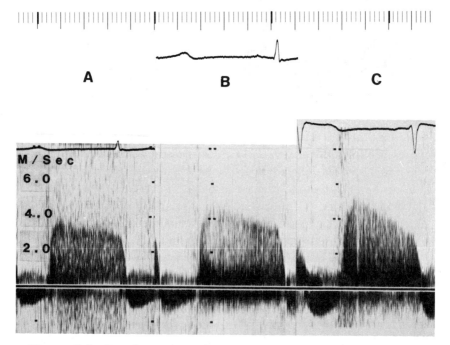

Figure 6.3 Panels A, B, and C show Doppler velocity spectral displays of aortic regurgitation recorded from the left ventrical apex view using continuous-wave Doppler enchocardiography. Note the difference in the slope of the velocity curves, indicating the speed with which the aortic-left ventricular pressure gradient decreases during diastole. The tracings were taken from patients with mild, moderate, and severe aortic regurgitation.

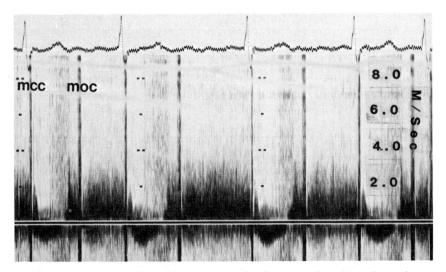

Figure 6.4 Doppler velocity record of an aortic regurgitant jet from a patient with a prosthetic mitral valve. Note that the aortic regurgitation starts before the mitral opening click, during the isometric relaxation period. moc, mitral opening click; mcc, mitral closing click.

end-diastolic pressure. The end-diastolic velocity should be used to calculate the left ventricular end-diastolic pressure. The end-diastolic velocities should be measured only from spectral displays showing blackening of the upper border until the very end of diastole (Fig. 6.2).

The slope of the velocity pattern from early to end-diastole is smooth and often reflects the severity of aortic regurgitation (Fig. 6.3). We have found that in severe aortic regurgitation it is steep, with a decrease in late diastolic velocities, whereas in mild cases there is little difference between the early and late-diastolic velocities. Mapping the left ventricular outflow tract using the pulsed Doppler sample volume has also been used for rough quantitation of the severity of aortic regurgitation. The sample volume is placed progressively farther in the left ventricle to determine how far from the aortic valve the regurgitant jet is sensed. It is assumed that a jet of mild aortic regurgitation will be localized to the left ventricular outflow space just below the aortic valve, whereas a jet of more severe regurgitation will be noted deeper in the left ventricular cavity. However, since the sample volume is placed

A   **B**

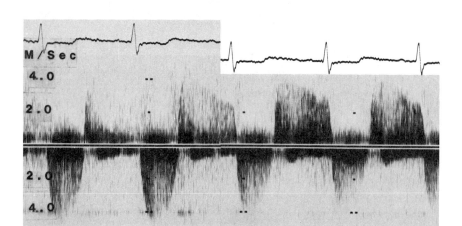

Figure 6.5 A continuous-wave Doppler transducer can be used to record the aortic stenotic and regurgitant jets simultaneously. However, the maximal velocity vectors of these two jets have different directions, so that different transducer angles are required to record the full spectrum of the velocity profile of the systolic and diastolic jets. Note that in panel A, when the aortic systolic velocity is fully profiled below the baseline, the regurgitant jet is not well received; the opposite is observed in panel B.

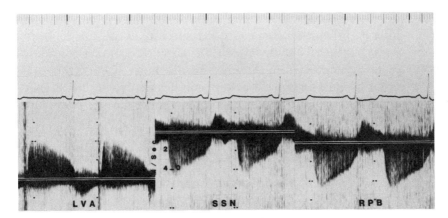

Figure 6.6   Doppler velocity spectral display of an aortic regurgitant jet recorded from the left ventricular apex (LVA), suprasternal notch (SSN), and right parasternal border (RPB). The best gray-scale display was obtained in records from the right parasternal border.

into the mid-left ventricle, the forward flow from the mitral valve will often be superimposed.

While using the continuous-wave Doppler technique for quantitation of the aortic regurgitant velocity profile, especially in patients with associated mitral stenosis, it is important to differentiate the abnormal velocity signals resulting from both lesions, since the spectral displays obtained from an apical transducer position are oriented in the same direction. However, aortic regurgitation starts in early diastole, during isovolumic relaxation (Fig. 6.4), whereas the mitral diastolic flow starts later, following mitral valve opening. This time difference tends to become shorter in the presence of severe mitral stenosis. Aortic regurgitation often has a velocity of more than 3.5 m/sec, which is not observed in patients with mitral stenosis.

While studying patients with combined aortic stenosis and regurgitation, one may obtain a record of both the forward and backward flows across the aortic valve from a single transducer position. However, it is important to recall that the maximal velocity vectors of these two jets may not be in the same axis and therefore should be mapped individually (Fig. 6.5). When one finds it difficult to obtain a good spectral display of the aortic regurgitant jet from the left ventricular apex, Doppler recordings *can* be attempted from the suprasternal notch or the right parasternal border. In some cases, it may be easy to record a good-quality Doppler tracing of the aortic regurgitant jet from all of these windows (Fig. 6.6).

7

DOPPLER EVALUATION OF TRICUSPID VALVE FUNCTION

The introduction of two-dimensional echocardiography has facilitated detailed imaging of the tricuspid valve and the right heart structures. The right ventricular apex view (right ventricular inflow view) images the right atrium, the tricuspid valve, and the right ventricular inflow portion. Primary pathology of the tricuspid valve may be evaluated by two-dimensional echocardiography. However, functional information on valvar stenosis and/or regurgitation is not quantifiable. Doppler evaluation of the flow through this valve would be ideal for the diagnosis and quantitation of tricuspid stenosis and/or tricuspid regurgitation even when they are associated with other valvar diseases.

The right ventricular apex view is obtained by placing the transducer midway between the left sternal border and the apex beat. It is directed anteriorly, cephalad, and to the right to image the right atrium and right ventricle. The tricuspid valve is imaged perpendicular to the axial plane. The Doppler beam is then positioned perpendicular to the tricuspid valve and parallel to the direction of blood flow across it. The sample volume is carefully placed on the right ventricular side of the tricuspid valve for measurement of diastolic blood flow through the valve (Fig. 7.1). When the two-dimensional image is frozen, a clear spectral display of the flow velocity pattern across the tricuspid valve may be obtained above the zero baseline. The audio output will give a low-pitched, rough diastolic noise. Once the wall motion filters, gray-scale compression, and reject modes are adjusted, a record can be obtained on a calibration scale of 0.2 or 0.5 m/sec/cm at a paper speed of 50 mm/sec. The normal flow pattern across the tricuspid valve resembles that across the mitral valve. Velocity rises to a peak in early diastole, during the rapid inflow phase to about 0.8 m/sec. It immediately comes down to near zero—reduced inflow—to rise again to about 0.5 m/sec during atrial systole. Maximum flow velocity varies from 0.5 to 0.8 m/sec. Blood flow velocity is low across the tricuspid valve because it has the largest dimension of all of the intracardiac valves. The maximum velocity often increases during inspiration due to increased flow.

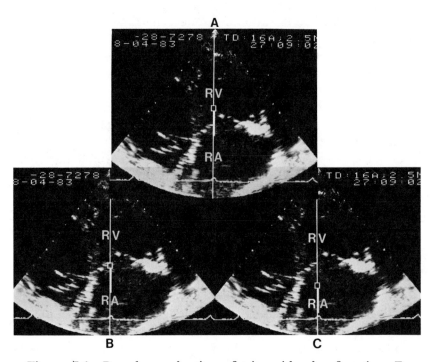

Figure 7.1 Doppler evaluation of tricuspid valve function. For measurement of diastolic flows and for assessment of tricuspid valve stenosis, the right ventricular apex view is imaged on the video screen and the sample volume is placed on the right ventricular side of the tricuspid orifice (panel A). For detection of tricuspid regurgitation, the sample volume is kept on the right atrial side of the tricuspid valve (panel B). The severity of tricuspid regurgitation is assessed by pulsed Doppler echo mapping of the right atrium. Generally, the presence of a regurgitation jet away from the valve (panel C) indicates a severe lesion. RV, right ventricle; RA, right atrium.

TRICUSPID STENOSIS

Tricuspid stenosis is commonly of rheumatic origin and often occurs with associated mitral and aortic valve disease. The presence of other diastolic murmurs, associated cardiac failure, and a low cardiac index may make the clinical diagnosis of tricuspid stenosis difficult. Even during cardiac catheterization, the utmost care is required to demonstrate the transtricuspid diastolic gradient. Unlike mitral stenosis, the diagnosis is confirmed by the demonstration of a small gradient. An end-diastolic gradient of 2 mm Hg across the tricuspid valve may indicate significant stenosis of the valve orifice. Narrowing of the tricuspid orifice increases the blood flow velocity, which can be estimated by placing the sample volume on the ventricular end of the tricuspid valve funnel. Doppler velocity tracings of diastolic flow across a stenosed tricuspid valve are easy to recognize because the mid-diastolic decrease in velocity is minimal. The increase in maximum velocity is only moderate. However, the velocity does not come down to normal at the end of diastole (Fig. 7.2). It may be about 0.75 m/sec or more. Such elevations in end-diastolic velocity can be better demonstrated when the recording is done while the breath is held at peak inspiration. It should be kept in mind that a large flow

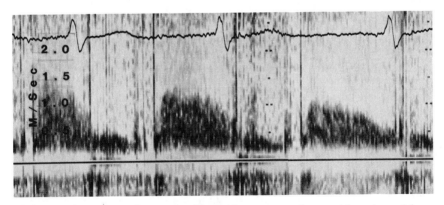

Figure 7.2 Doppler recordings from a patient with tricuspid valve obstruction. Note that even though the maximum velocity is only 1.25 m/sec, it remains high until the end of diastole.

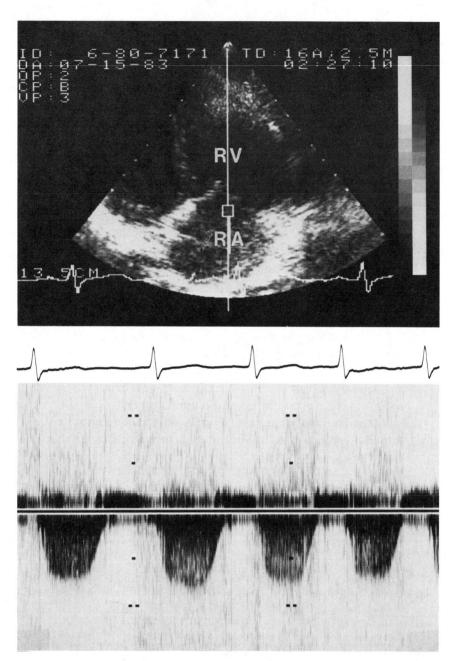

Figure 7.3 The pulsed Doppler technique can be used to detect tricuspid regurgitation (upper panel). However, for measurement of maximal velocity of the regurgitant jet (lower panel), a contin-

through the tricuspid valve in atrial septal defect, an anomalous pulmonary venous connection, or anemia may also increase the maximal velocity of flow. However, in these situations, the velocity returns to normal at the end of diastole.

TRICUSPID REGURGITATION

Tricuspid regurgitation is often "functional," secondary to pulmonary hypertension or chronic right ventricular failure. It may also result from a primary disease of the tricuspid valve such as infective endocarditis, carcinoid syndrome, or Ebstein's anomaly. Tricuspid regurgitation is often difficult to diagnose, and its severity is even harder to quantitate. Contrast echocardiography is reported to be a reliable method for the confirmation of tricuspid regurgitation. Besides being nonquantitative, it requires peripheral venous injections of a saline or dextrose solution. The Doppler examination of the right atrium can easily diagnose tricuspid regurgitation with a high degree of accuracy.

The right ventricular apex view is imaged on the video screen, and the Doppler sample volume is placed on the right atrial side of the tricuspid valve (Fig. 7.1*b*, *c*). When tricuspid reflux is present, the audio output will give a medium- or high-pitched systolic whistling noise. As the regurgitant jet is directed away from the transducer, the spectral display will appear below the baseline (Fig. 7.3). Hence, the baseline may be raised to the top of the screen. Once the two-dimensional echo image is frozen, the calibration factor should be adjusted and the wall motion artifact filters and reject set so that the full-velocity spectral display is clearly visible. When tricuspid regurgitation is severe, it is easily

uous-wave or extended pulsed Doppler facility is required, since the velocity measured is often more than 2 m/sec. When the peak velocity is accurately recorded, it is possible to estimate right ventricular systolic pressure (see text). RV, right ventricle; RA, right atrium.

picked up and the respiratory increase in velocity is easily demonstrable. However, the changes in the direction of the Doppler beam that occur with deep inspiration can make the latter maneuver difficult.

The spectral display of the velocity profile of tricuspid regurgitation starts immediately after the QRS complex and comes down at the end of systole. The velocity generally varies between 2.5 and 4.0 m/sec. Primary tricuspid regurgitation occurs with a low velocity that decreases after mid-systole. The velocity of the regurgitant jet represents the pressure difference between the right ventricle (RV) and the right atrium (RA) during systole. It could be used to calculate the systolic RV-RA pressure gradient using the formula $\Delta P = V^2 \times 4$. When this pressure gradient is known, it can be used to calculate the right ventricular systolic pressure. The right atrial pressure may be estimated as the systolic jugular venous pressure (plus 5 cm as the jugular venous pressure is measured from the sternal angle). Adding the right atrial pressure to the systolic RV-RA gradient will give the right ventricular systolic pressure.

The severity of tricuspid regurgitation can also be judged by Doppler mapping of the right atrium. The sample volume is systematically placed away from the tricuspid valve to find out how far in the right atrium the regurgitant jet is picked up. Only when the regurgitation is significant can it be picked up away from the tricuspid valve. In severe tricuspid regurgitation, the systolic reflux of blood toward the right atrium can be picked up even on the right ventricular side of the tricuspid valve. Mild tricuspid regurgitation is a common finding without associated murmur even in an otherwise normal heart.

Velocity of TR = RV - RA

Pk pressure of TR = RV - 14

∴ Pk press of TR + 14 = RV = Pul wedge press

8

DOPPLER EVALUATION OF PULMONARY VALVE FUNCTION

The pulmonary area over the precordium is a common location of innocent systolic murmurs or of murmurs due to right ventricular outflow obstruction or ventricular septal defects. Doppler examinations can be effectively used for the differential diagnosis of these lesions, as well as for quantitation of the obstruction at any level in the right ventricular outflow tract. It is most useful in ruling out significant heart disease in patients who have innocent systolic murmurs in the pulmonary area.

The pulmonary valve with the right ventricular outflow tract and main pulmonary artery can be imaged near the axial plane in the parasternal short-axis view. This procedure facilitates Doppler studies of flow velocities in relation to this valve. For placement of the Doppler beam perpendicular to the pulmonary valve and parallel to the main pulmonary artery, a movable cursor of the Doppler beam is helpful. Many Doppler echo machines are provided with this facility. Since the Doppler studies are done in the near field, it is useful to obtain a clear, magnified image of the outflow of the right ventricle and the main pulmonary artery. It may be preferable to use a 3.5- or 5.0-MHz two-dimensional echocardiographic transducer for this purpose.

For measurement of flow velocity across the pulmonary valve, the sample volume is placed immediately in front of the pulmonary valve in the main pulmonary artery (Fig. 8.1). The audio output will give a rough, short sound during systole, and the spectral display will show the velocity profile of the forward flow below the baseline, since the blood flow is away from the transducer. Once the wall motion filters, calibration, and reject modes are properly adjusted, a record can be obtained at paper speeds of 50 and 100 mm/sec. The spectral display will show a pattern similar to that of the aortic flow velocity, starting early in systole, immediately reaching a sharp peak, and coming down to the baseline toward the end of systole. The maximum velocity varies from 0.6 to 1.1 m/sec (mean, 0.75 m/sec). The velocity of blood flow across the pulmonary valve increases during increased flow due to left-to-right shunts, hyperdynamic circulatory states, and pulmonary stenosis. Measurement of blood flow velocity across the main pulmonary artery and the calculated cross-sectional area of the latter are used to calculate pulmonary blood flow in patients with

85

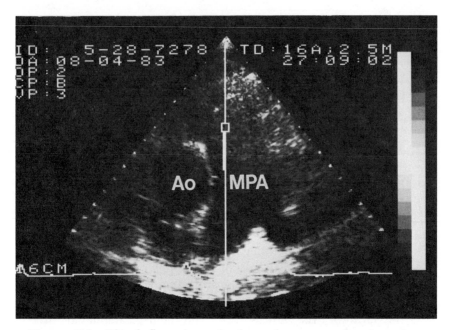

Figure 8.1 Blood flow through the pulmonary valve into the main pulmonary artery is measured by imaging the right ventricular outflow tract, pulmonary valve, and main pulmonary artery in the parasternal short-axis view. The sample volume is placed in the main pulmonary artery (MPA) in front of the pulmonary valve. For measuring velocity vectors in patients with pulmonary stenosis, a similar technique using the continuous-wave Doppler technique is employed. Ao, aorta.

left-to-right shunts. The systemic:pulmonary flow ratio can be calculated when the systemic flow is also estimated from aortic flow velocity and the cross-sectional area of the ascending aorta.

PULMONARY STENOSIS

Right ventricular outflow obstruction at various levels from the low infundibulum to the main pulmonary artery is the common denominator in many congenital cyanotic heart diseases. The technique of diagnosing and quantitating pulmonary stenosis is dealt with in detail in Chapter 11.

Often the obstruction at the right ventricular outflow may be infundibular or may occur at many levels. The site of obstruction can be located by pulsed Doppler mapping. The sample volume is placed serially from the proximal part of the right ventricular outflow to the bifurcation point of the main pulmonary artery for the detection of high-velocity jets. Jets can be identified by the sudden appearance of aliasing. At the site of aliasing, the maximum velocity of the jet is measured using the extended pulsed Doppler or continuous-wave Doppler technique. However, it is very difficult to obtain a clear image of the right ventricular infundibular region in patients with congenital cyanotic heart diseases such as tetralogy of Fallot. When a clear image is obtained, it may be impossible to image the infundibular region parallel to the Doppler beam, since the former is nearly always perpendicular to the axial plane in the two-dimensional echo image.

PULMONARY REGURGITATION

Pulmonary regurgitation as an organic valvar lesion is uncommon. It can occur as an isolated congenital abnormality or along with tetralogy of Fallot. However, it is more commonly found secondary to severe pulmonary hypertension in atrial septal defect, patent ductus arteriosis, or rheumatic mitral stenosis. It can also occur after infective endocarditis or after surgical procedures in the right ventricular outflow tract. The murmur of pulmonary regurgitation starts after the pulmonary second sound and lasts for varying periods in diastole. Since it is audible in the pulmonary area and the left parasternal border, it is difficult to differentiate it from the murmur of aortic regurgitation. Linear contrast echocardiography is widely used to demonstrate regurgitation across the pulmonary valve. Doppler echocardiography is equally sensitive and totally noninvasive for the above purpose.

The right ventricular outflow tract, pulmonary valve, and main pulmonary artery are imaged as described earlier. The Doppler

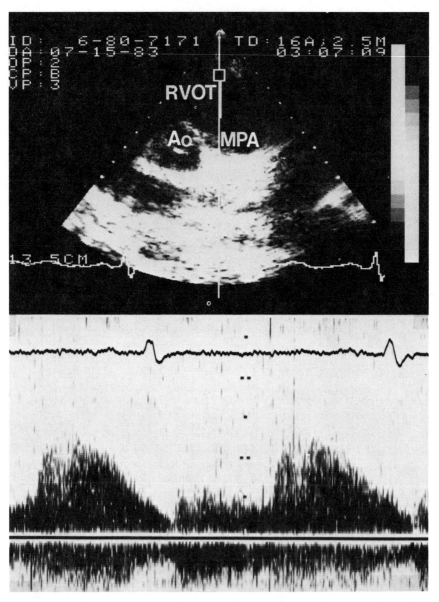

Figure 8.2 Pulmonary regurgitation recorded from a patient without pulmonary hypertension. Note the rapid reduction in velocity and the absence of an end-diastolic gradient from the pulmonary artery to the right ventricle. RVOT, right ventricular outflow tract; MPA, main pulmonary artery; Ao, aorta.

beam is kept perpendicular to the pulmonary valve and the sample volume below it in the right ventricular outflow region. Pulmonary regurgitation is manifested as a diastolic hissing noise in the audio output. Once the image is frozen, one can see the spectral display of the regurgitant jet throughout diastole above the baseline. Once the wall motion filters, reject mode, and calibration are adjusted, the display should be recorded on strip chart. It will show maximum velocity of the regurgitant jet in early diastole. When it is associated with pulmonary hypertension, the velocity may remain high throughout diastole. In isolated, nonpulmonary hypertensive pulmonary regurgitation, the velocity decreases rapidly as diastole progresses and may reach the baseline (Fig. 8.2). The velocity of the regurgitant jet is only about 1–2 m/sec when it is not associated with pulmonary hypertension. One can attempt to quantitate the severity of pulmonary regurgitation by mapping the right ventricular outflow tract using the Doppler sample volume. The object is to determine how far away from the pulmonary valve in the right ventricular outflow region the regurgitant jet can be sensed. Only severe pulmonary regurgitation can be detected in the lower infundibular region.

It is important to remember that if the Doppler beam is directed laterally and anteriorly in relation to the pulmonary valve, the blood flow through the anterior descending branch of the left coronary artery can give an early diastolic velocity spectral display above the baseline. However, this direction of angulation gives a pattern similar to the normal systolic flow pattern, with a narrow band of frequencies, and can be recorded only from a very narrow zone in the echo image.

DIAGNOSIS OF PULMONARY HYPERTENSION FROM DOPPLER VELOCITY RECORDINGS

In discussing the usefulness of quantitating the tricuspid regurgitation jet velocity, it was mentioned that this value reflects the pressure difference between the right ventricle and right atrium.

From the maximum velocity of the tricuspid regurgitation jet, one can calculate the systolic gradient from the right ventricle to the right atrium. The height of the jugular venous pressure measured clinically, when added to the calculated RV-RA systolic gradient, will give the right ventricular systolic pressure and hence the pulmonary artery systolic pressure. In patients with ventricular septal defect in which flow velocity across the defect can be measured, it may be used to calculate the pressure difference (gradient) between the left and right ventricles. Left ventricular systolic pressure can be estimated by the sphygmamonometer as the systolic blood pressure. Subtracting the LV-RV pressure gradient from the systolic blood pressure will give the right ventricular

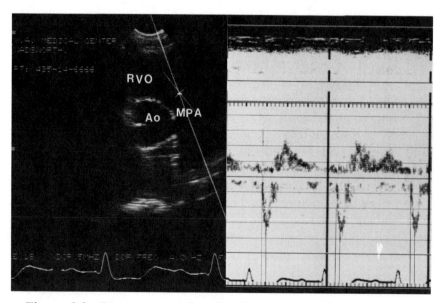

Figure 8.3   Pumonary acceleration line recorded from a patient with primary pulmonary hypertension. The two-dimensional echo picture demonstrates the direction of the Doppler beam and the sample volume in the main pulmonary artery (MPA). The Doppler beam is 15° tangential to the direction of blood flow. The Doppler velocity display shows a pulmonary acceleration line of 0.05 sec, indicating pulmonary hypertension. RVO, right ventricular outflow; Ao, aorta.

systolic pressure (or the pulmonary artery pressure in the absence of associated pulmonic stenosis). Hatle and Angelsen (1982) used the pulmonary valve closure (Pc) to tricuspid valve opening time (To) (Pc-To interval) to calculate the pulmonary artery pressure. Valve closure and opening times were measured from simultaneous Doppler velocity and phonocardiographic recordings. The Pc-To interval was 10–50 msec in normal subjects and appeared to be more than 50 msec in patients with pulmonary hypertension. Pulmonary artery pressure could be assessed from the Pc-To interval, which increases proportionately with pulmonary artery pressure and inversely with heart rate. Interested readers may refer to a table provided by Burstein (*Br. Heart J* 29:396–404, 1967).

Recently, many workers have noticed shortening of the pulmonary artery velocity acceleration time in patients with pulmonary hypertension. The pulmonary acceleration time is the interval from the beginning of the Doppler velocity display to its peak. Normally, it is 137 ± 24 msec. It is shortened in patients with pulmonary hypertension to 97 ± 20 msec (Kitabatake 1983). A pulmonary hypertension in most patients (Fig. 8.3). Pulmonary artery acceleration time estimated by Doppler echocardiography is inversely related to increasing mean pulmonary artery pressure. Mahan and co-workers (1983) recently demonstrated that the pulmonary acceleration time is linearly related to the mean pulmonary artery pressure and showed that the latter could be calculated using the following formula:

$$\text{Mean PAP} = (-0.45)(\text{PAT}) + 79$$

where PAP represents the pulmonary artery pressure and PAT is the pulmonary acceleration time. These recent observations await further confirmation by independent investigators.

normal pul ace time $= 137 \pm 24$ *msec*

PAH $= 97 \pm 20$ *msec*

9

DOPPLER EVALUATION OF PROSTHETIC HEART VALVES

Ever since the introduction of prosthetic heart valve replacement surgery, long-term functional and structural evaluation of the replaced valve has been unsatisfactory. Noninvasive procedures such as M-mode and two-dimensional echocardiography, echophonocardiography, and cinefluoroscopy have been used for this purpose, but without uniform success. Detailed echocardiographic visualization of various components of a mechanical prosthesis is difficult due to the high echo reflectivity of prosthetic valve materials. Multiple reverberations and acoustic shadowing distort the image of the valve, and especially the area behind it. In porcine xenografts, imaging of the valve leaflets is generally possible. It has been suggested that measurement of flow characteristics across the prosthetic valve using Doppler echocardiography can periodically assess the functional characteristics of these valves. Our early experience indicates that the combined use of two-dimensional echo and Doppler techniques is invaluable for structural and functional assessment of prosthetic valves.

ASSESSMENT OF PROSTHETIC MITRAL VALVE FUNCTIONS

The technique of measuring Doppler flow velocity across a prosthetic mitral valve is similar to that used under normal circumstances. The left ventricle, the mitral valve, and the left atrium are imaged from the left ventricular apex. The Doppler beam is directed perpendicular to the plane of the mitral valve and parallel to the direction of blood flow. The sample volume can be easily placed on the left ventricular side of porcine heterograft valves to measure blood flow velocity. However, in patients with a mechanical prosthesis such as the Starr-Edwards valve, this procedure may be difficult in view of the dense echoes seen behind the valve. Moreover, the maximal velocity vectors are often on either side of the valve orifice. Careful mapping of the entire width of the valve orifice, as well as placement of the sample volume distal to the valve cage, are important in obtaining a good-quality Doppler recording. In evaluating the St. Jude's prosthesis, the sample volume can be easily threaded through the valve orifice because of its central flow pattern. Holen and colleagues (1977) have found it easy to measure the flow characteristics across the Bjork-Shiley valve, possibly because a number of jets issue from the valve in different directions. Flow patterns across the Lillehei-Kastor valve have shown four major diverging jets. Hence, the Doppler beam can be aligned parallel to any of them.

Normally functioning prosthetic valves produce loud opening and closing clicks, which may be also useful as time markers in the Doppler recordings (Fig. 9.1). The early diastolic and atrial systolic increase in flow velocity and the characteristic M-shaped

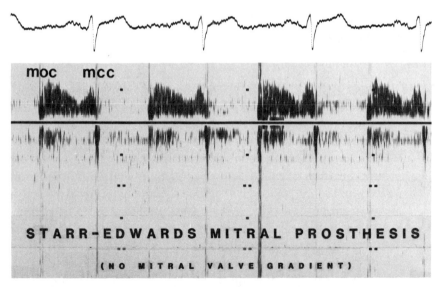

Figure 9.1 Doppler velocity recording of diastolic flow through a normally functioning Starr-Edwards mitral prosthesis. Note the loud mitral opening (moc) and closing (mcc) clicks.

flow pattern across the mitral valve are generally retained across the prosthetic valves. However, the mean and maximum flow velocities are higher than those found in the normal mitral valve. Weinstein (1983), in a study of flow velocities through the St. Jude's mitral prosthesis, found that the mean and maximum velocities were 0.73 ± 0.16 and 1.38 ± 0.33 m/sec (normal values, 0.35 ± 0.06 and 0.78 ± 0.02 m/sec), respectively. However, an increase in end-diastolic velocity was not observed in a normally functioning prosthesis. When this finding is present, it reflects a persistent pressure gradient between the left atrium and the left ventricle at end diastole and is indicative of prosthetic valve obstruction.

A decrease in the flow velocity profile during the first half of diastole can be used to estimate the pressure half-time (see Chapter 3). Hatle and Angelsen (1982) noted a slight increase in atrioventricular pressure half-time (or gradient) across the prosthetic mitral valve. The pressure half-time may not be used for accurate calculation of the effective valve orifice area in some normally functioning prosthetic valves, since this formula does not hold good for valves with larger cross-sectional orifice areas.

Narrowing of the prosthetic mitral valve orifice is generally easy to assess. It is indicated by an increase in maximum, mean, and end-diastolic Doppler flow velocities across the mitral orifice. Continuous-wave or extended pulsed Doppler echocardiography should be used for accurate measurement of such velocities. Under such circumstances, atrioventricular pressure half-time can be estimated, and the value obtained can be used to calculate the mitral valve area. Since the maximum flow velocity as measured by the Doppler echo technique cannot be overestimated, the severity of obstruction will not be overestimated. Mitral regurgitation through a malfunctioning prosthetic valve or through the paravalvar region is observed more often than valve narrowing. Such mitral regurgitant jets may be inaudible during routine auscultation. Even when they are audible, it is difficult to assess the severity of regurgitation clinically. Doppler mapping on the left atrial side of the mitral valve can easily pick up some regurgitant jets (Fig. 9.2). It should be remembered that prosthetic valve regurgitation often occurs through the paravalvar regions, which are generally eccentric. The sample volume should be systemati-

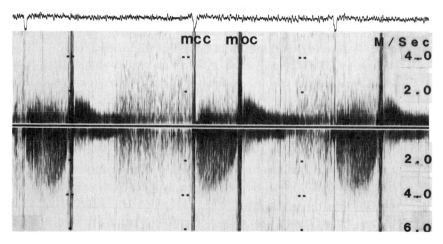

Figure 9.2   Paravalvar mitral regurgitation recorded from a patient with a Bjork-Shiley mitral valve. Note the prominent mitral opening (moc) and closing clicks (mcc).

cally placed from the aortic end to the left border of the left atrium. When a regurgitant jet is sensed, the velocity and the full profile should be carefully measured using continuous-wave or extended pulsed wave Doppler technique. Some workers have attempted to place sample volumes more distally from the mitral valve to detect how far away in the left atrium a regurgitant jet can be recorded. This procedure may give a rough assessment of the severity of the mitral regurgitation. Differentiation of mitral valve obstruction from aortic regurgitation and of mitral regurgitation from aortic valve obstruction was described in earlier chapters.

ASSESSMENT OF PROSTHETIC AORTIC VALVE FUNCTIONS

Measurement of blood flow velocity in the aortic root is technically more difficult in patients with prosthetic aortic valves than in normal adult subjects. The Starr-Edwards and Bjork-Shiley valves produce alterations in flow patterns in the ascending aorta. Hence, Doppler flow velocity should always be measured systematically from the left ventricular apex, suprasternal notch, and right parasternal border, and only the technically best records should be analyzed to judge flow characteristics across the valve. Continuous-wave or extended pulsed wave Doppler technique will always be required for measurement of maximum systolic blood flow velocity across the aortic valve. The velocity profile characteristics are similar to those of a normal native valve. Doppler tracings from patients with prosthetic valves can be easily identified because of the loud opening and closing clicks. As observed in patients

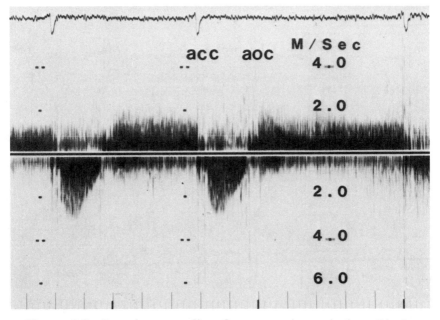

Figure 9.3 Doppler recording from a patient wiwth a Bjork-Shiley aortic valve. Abnormal diastolic velocities indicate aortic regurgitation. Since the Doppler beam could not be placed parallel to the maximal velocity vectors of the aortic regurgitant jet, only part of the spectrum of regurgitant velocity is seen above the baseline. The aortic systolic velocity seen below the baseline shows a velocity of 3 m/sec, indicating a mild residual gradient.

with prosthetic mitral valves, the maximum and mean velocities are higher than those seen in normal, healthy subjects with native valves. Weinstein and colleagues (1983) reported mean and maximum systolic flow velocities across the St. Judes prosthesis of 1.23 ± 0.25 and 1.97 ± 0.52, respectively, whereas normal, healthy native valves showed mean and maximum flow velocities of only 0.89 ± 0.14 and 1.22 ± 0.19, respectively. The values for other types of prosthetic valves without central flow patterns may be higher. A high-velocity flow across an obstructed prosthetic aortic valve has all of the characteristics of valvar aortic stenosis. The maximum and mean velocities are more than 2.5 m/sec, and the peak velocity is reached later in systole. One of the main advantages of Doppler echocardiography is its ability to pick up even mild

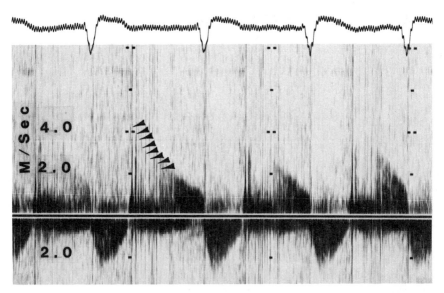

Figure 9.4 Doppler evaluation is often useful in assessing the functional characteristics of prosthetic heart valves. This patient has a porcine aortic valve dysfunction due to prolapse of the cusps into the left ventricular outflow tract. Note the multiple clicking sounds produced by vibrations of the prolapsing cusp and associated aortic regurgitation. An estimated systolic gradient of 25 mm Hg is present.

aortic regurgitation, which is often inaudible (Fig. 9.3). This regurgitation may be an early indication of prosthetic valve dysfunction. In patients with a porcine aortic valve, periodic evaluation for aortic regurgitation has been used to indicate valve dysfunction secondary to cusp degeneration. Aortic regurgitation can also be secondary to infection of the prosthetic valve. A badly damaged or torn cusp of a heterograft valve may vibrate in diastole, and the Doppler recording may show characteristic multiple clicking noises in Doppler tracings (Fig. 9.4).

10

QUANTITATION OF BLOOD FLOW USING DOPPLER ECHOCARDIOGRAPHY

Two-dimensional echocardiographic Doppler equipment capable of imaging both cardiac structures and flow velocities is well suited to measure the volume of blood flow. With a knowledge of the cross-sectional area of a vessel, or an orifice through which the flow is occurring and the velocity of flow, the volume of flow can be calculated using the formula

$$\text{Volume } (Q) = \text{area (cm}^2) \times \text{velocity (cm/sec)}$$
$$\times \text{ duration of ejection (sec)} \times \text{heart rate}$$

Using this formula, blood flow through various cardiac valves and great vessels may be calculated. Once the diameter (D) of a circular structure such as the aorta is measured from the two-dimensional echo image, its cross-sectional area may be calculated using the formula Area $= \pi(\frac{1}{2} \cdot D)^2$. For all volumetric calculations of flow in systole, the mean velocity is used. The instantaneous velocity measured every 40 msec is averaged to obtain the mean systolic velocity in centimeters per second. Ideally, the mean velocity should be the mean velocity in the cross-sectional area (space-averaged velocity). In blood vessels, the velocity of the blood flow varies across the lumen due to viscous friction between the vessel wall and the blood. The velocity is maximum in the center of the vessel and near zero at the periphery. During systolic ejection, the velocity profile tends to be flatter. In the aorta and the pulmonary artery, where the blood flow is strongly pulsatile, the systolic velocity profile is fairly flat; hence, a time-averaged mean velocity can be used for the calculation of stroke volume.

CALCULATION OF CARDIAC OUTPUT [SYSTEMIC FLOW (Qs)] FROM AORTIC FLOW VELOCITY

The calculation of cardiac output from aortic flow velocity is a commonly used approach. The ascending aorta is imaged from the suprasternal notch, and the Doppler sample volume is placed in the ascending aorta above the level of the sinuses of Valsalva. Aortic flow velocity is the measured. Care must be taken to maintain an intercept angle (cosine Θ) of less than 15° and to obtain the full systolic velocity recording during each cardiac cycle. The diameter of the aorta in systole is measured at the point where the sample volume is placed from a printout of the two-dimensional echo picture. Alternatively, an M-mode and/or two-dimensional echo picture of the aorta can be obtained from the parasternal long-axis view for measurement of the aortic diameter. The cross-sectional area of the ascending aorta and the mean systolic velocity are calculated and used to determine systemic flow using the formula mentioned earlier. It is important to remember that the aortic diameter and the aortic flow velocity should be measured at the same point in the aorta.

MITRAL VALVE ORIFICE METHOD FOR CALCULATION OF CARDIAC OUTPUT

The mitral orifice can be imaged clearly in the parasternal short-axis view. Valdes-Cruz, et al (1983) used an effective mean diastolic cross-sectional orifice area of the mitral valve to calculate the stroke volume. The maximum mitral valve area is obtained by planimetering the orifice area from a two-dimensional short-axis view. From the above view, a cursor-derived M-mode scan is also recorded at a paper speed of 100 mm/sec. Maximum mitral valve leaflet separation is measured at the E point in the M-mode tracing. The mean mitral leaflet separation is calculated by averaging the mitral leaflet separations every 0.04 sec in diastole. Multiplying the maximal mitral valve orifice area by the ratio of mean to maximal mitral valve leaflet separation gives the effective mean diastolic cross-sectional mitral orifice area. Mitral diastolic flow is recorded from the left ventricular apical view using the pulsed Doppler technique at a paper speed of 100 mm/sec. The sample volume is kept at the mitral orifice in the left ventricle, and the Doppler beam is parallel to the transmitral flow. Mean mitral flow velocity in diastole is calculated by planimetering the area under the velocity trace and time averaging. Cardiac output (CO) is calculated using the formula

$$CO = \frac{\text{mean velocity} \times \text{effective mean mitral valve area} \times 60}{\text{Cos } \Theta}$$

where Cos Θ is equal to 1. This method has recently been simplified using the maximum diastolic mitral annulus diameter measured from the apical four-chamber view. A circular fixed flow area is calculated from the annulus diameter and is used instead of the effective mean mitral valve area. A similar approach using the tricuspid annulus permits estimation of systemic venous return or flow across the tricuspid orifice.

ESTIMATION OF PULMONARY BLOOD (Qp)

Quantitation of pulmonary blood flow is important in many patients with intracardiac shunts. The reliability of Doppler estimates of pulmonary flow has been demonstrated in many congenital heart diseases. The technique is similar to that employed for estimation of the systemic blood flow. The pulmonary artery is imaged in the parasternal short-axis view. Since the main pulmonary artery is dilated and superficial, it may be easy to image it in children with left-to-right shunts. Once the pulmonary valve and main pulmonary artery are clearly visualized, the pulsed Doppler sample volume is placed in the proximal main pulmonary artery and the Doppler beam is aligned parallel to the direction of blood flow. The velocity profile of pulmonary flow in systole is recorded over several cardiac cycles, and the mean systolic velocity is estimated. The diameter of the main pulmonary artery where the Doppler sample volume was placed is measured from the two-dimensional echo picture and the cross-sectional area calculated. Flow through the main pulmonary artery is calculated using the formula Area (cm^2) × velocity (cm/sec) × duration of ejection (sec) × heart rate.

CALCULATION OF LEFT-TO-RIGHT SHUNTS

Atrial Septal Defect

Since the left-to-right shunt occurs at the atrial level, flow through the dilated main pulmonary artery is fairly smooth and Doppler velocity profiling is easy. Hence, pulmonary flow can be calculated from the pulmonary artery flow velocity and the cross-sectional area. Systemic flow can be estimated from the ascending aorta or the mitral valve orifice. It is easier to image the ascending aorta in children from the suprasternal notch so that aortic flow can be estimated easily.

Ventricular Septal Defect

Defects in the interventricular septum are common in the upper part of the septum, often close to the outflow tract of the right ventricle. The systolic jet of blood coming through the ventricular septal defect thus produces turbulence in the outflow tract of the right ventricle and the pulmonary artery. Hence, one may find it difficult to get good-quality Doppler velocity recordings from the main pulmonary artery in these patients. However, all of the pulmonary flow eventually must pass through the mitral valve, and flow calculated using the mitral orifice method will represent the pulmonary flow in patients with ventricular septal defect. Systemic flow can be estimated from the ascending aorta, as described earlier.

Patent Ductus Arteriosus

A left-to-right shunt across a patent ductus arteriosus alters the flow patterns in the pulmonary arteries. The systemic venous return reaches the right ventricle and is pumped into the main pulmonary artery. At the same time, shunted blood coming across the ductus enters the proximal part of the left pulmonary artery. Consequent turbulent flow in the main pulmonary artery makes it difficult to obtain good velocity records of pulmonary artery flow. However, all of the pulmonary flow has to cross the mitral valve (and aortic valve); hence, it can be calculated using the mitral orifice method. Since aortic flow also represents the total left ventricular output, which includes the left-to-right shunt, the systemic venous flow measured at the tricuspid orifice or the right ventricular outflow tract is used to quantitate systemic flow. Although quantitative evaluation of systemic and pulmonary blood flow is often possible, the reported studies show that even when an absolute measure of flow by Doppler techniques is not correlated with indicator dilution techniques, the change in flow in a given patient correlates well by both methods.

ESTIMATION OF REGURGITANT VOLUME

In patients with mitral regurgitation, part of the blood passes into the left atrium while systolic ejection into the aorta takes place. In diastole, the pulmonary venous return and the regurgitant fraction pass into the left ventricle through the mitral valve; these flows can be estimated using the mitral orifice method. Systemic flow can be calculated from the ascending aorta using the suprasternal approach. The mitral regurgitant volume is obtained by subtracting the aortic systolic flow from the mitral diastolic flow during each cardiac cycle. Similarly, the aortic regurgitant volume can be calculated by subtracting the mitral diastolic flow from the aortic systolic flow measured at the level of the ascending aorta. However, the feasibility of this method has not been adequately tested.

11

DOPPLER EXAMINATION OF COMMON CONGENITAL CARDIAC DEFECTS

Two-dimensional echocardiography has allowed diagnostic non-invasive visualization of most congenital heart lesions. However, small defects, particularly in the atrial or ventricular septa, have been difficult to visualize confidently. Furthermore, patent ductus arteriosus, coarctation, and mild pulmonary valve stenosis have been difficult to diagnose or quantify in terms of severity. In these circumstances, Doppler echocardiography plays an important complementary role. The technique of the examination and the characteristic spectral flow patterns of common congenital cardiac defects are presented.

ATRIAL SEPTAL DEFECT

The noninvasive diagnosis of atrial septal defect has been greatly facilitated by two-dimensional echocardiography.[1] However, documentation of left-to-right shunting has required peripheral venous contrast echocardiography[2] or cardiac catheterization. A pulsed Doppler ultrasonic examination directed at the atrial septum allows detection and/or confirmation of left-to-right shunting in the majority of patients with atrial septal defect.[3,4] Ideally, the transducer placed in the subcostal position, and the beam is directed toward the atrial septum. The pulsed Doppler examination is performed by placing the sample volume in the right atrium adjacent to the fossa ovalis. In a patient with atrial septal defect, pulsed Doppler echocardiography reveals a characteristic audio and spectral pattern (Fig. 11.1). Since the left-to-right shunt flow

This chapter was written by Mark J. Callahan, M.D., Consultant in Cardiovascular Diseases and Internal Medicine, Assistant Professor of Medicine, Mayo Medical School; James B. Seward, M.D., Consultant in Cardiovascular Diseases, Internal Medicine and Pediatric Cardiology, and Associate Professor of Medicine and Pediatrics, Mayo Medical School; and A. Jamil Tajik, M.D., Consultant in Cardiovascular Diseases, Internal Medicine and Pediatric Cardiology and Professor of Medicine, Mayo Medical School, Director of Echocardiography Laboratory, Mayo Clinic, Rochester, Minnesota.

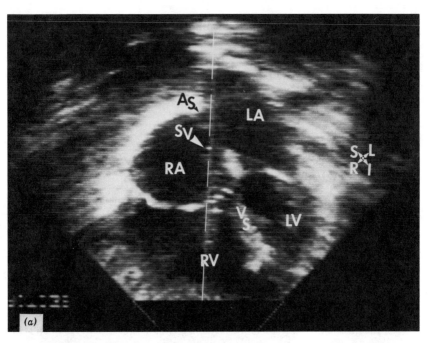

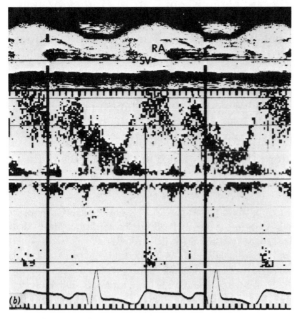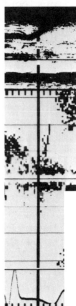

is toward the transducer, the spectral signal is displayed above the velocity baseline. The flow pattern consists of a low-velocity, "turbulent" wave commencing in late systole and continuing through diastole. Velocity diminishes in mid-diastole and is accentuated with atrial systole. Although this pattern was first described using an intracardiac Doppler probe,[5] transcutaneous two-dimensional echo-guided pulsed Doppler examinations yield the same characteristic profile. A very brief systolic right-to-left flow with velocities in an opposite (negative) direction may be seen during the isovolumic contraction period in some patients.

In patients in whom subcostal imaging is of suboptimal quality, pulsed Doppler examination of the atrial septum using a low parasternal or apical four-chamber view can yield a similar diagnostic spectral pattern. In patients suspected of having atrial septal defect in whom a defect cannot be directly visualized by two-dimensional echocardiography, pulsed Doppler examination of the entire atrial septum should be methodically undertaken.

Doppler quantitation of the shunt volume is promising. Doppler measurements of pulmonary-to-systemic flow ratios have been performed in patients with intracardiac shunts.[6] However, this technique is yet to be tested clinically in a large group of patients.

Figure 11.1 (*a*)Atrial Septal Defect. Left: Two-dimensional echocardiogram in the four-chamber plane (apex oriented downward) illustrating the sample volume (SV) position used during pulsed wave Doppler assessment of atrial septal defect. Note that the SV is positioned in the right atrium (RA) adjacent to the suspected defect. As, atrial septum; LA, left atrium; LV = left ventricle; RV = right ventricle; L = left; I = inferior; R = right; S = superior. (*b*) *Right:* Pulsed Doppler spectral output showing the charactristic flow pattern of the left-to-right shunt across an atrial septal defect. Note that the positive spectral deflection begins in late systole, is present throughout diastole, and is accentuated in atrial systole, SV, sample volume; RA, right atrium. Arrows illustrate the relationship of the spectral output of the electrocardiographic timing of the cardiac cycle.

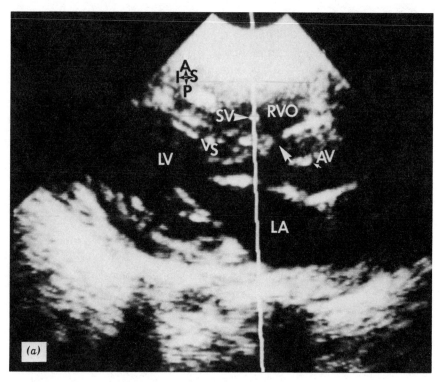

Figure 11.2 Ventricular septal defect. (*a*) *Left:* Two-Dimensional echocardiographic parasternal long-axis view of the left ventricle. The sample volume (SV) is placed in the right ventricular outflow tract (RVO). The SV is placed over a suspected ventricular septal defect (arrow). AV, aortic valve; LA, left atrium; LV, left ventricle; P, posterior; I, inferior; A, anterior; S, superior. (*b*) *Right:* Pulsed Doppler spectral pattern consistent with a ventricular septal defect. The SV is in the RVO. Note that there is a "turbulent" spectral disturbance during ventricular systole. This disturbance is characteristic of a high velocity across the ventricular septal defect, which produces aliasing (foldover) of the Doppler signal. The spectral disturbance seen during diastole is characteristic of cardiac wall or valve motion.

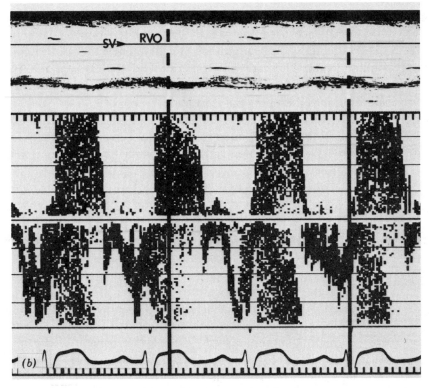

Figure 11.2 (*continued*)

VENTRICULAR SEPTAL DEFECT

The diagnosis of ventricular septal defect by two-dimensional echocardiography can be enhanced by the use of Doppler echocardiography.[7] A complete assessment begins with a detailed two-dimensional echocardiographic examination of the ventricular septum for detection and localization of the ventricular septal defect. Paramembranous defects 3 mm or more in diameter can be confidently visualized. Pulsed Doppler echocardiography is used for confirmation of left-to-right shunting by placing the sample volume in the right ventricle adjacent to the suspected or visible defect.

The characteristic pulsed Doppler spectral pattern is a pansystolic turbulence accompanied by an audible shunt signal (Fig. 11.2). Alterations of beam direction will optimize the spectral and audible signal. The high-velocity jet of a ventricular septal defect will frequently be transmitted to the right ventricular outflow tract and even into the pulmonary artery.

Small defects in the apical trabecular septum can be difficult to diagnose by two-dimensional imaging alone. In these situations, the pulsed Doppler examination is extremely helpful. Apical and subcostal views of the trabecular septum are obtained, and the sample volume is placed near the right ventricular apex. The sample volume is moved along the right septal surface to detect a systolic high-velocity, turbulent flow. Left-to-right shunt flow across a ventricular septal defect is directed toward the transducer and appears as a positive deflection on the spectral display (Fig. 11.2).

If the right ventricular pressure is normal, the jet will be of high velocity, and frequency aliasing will be noted in the pulsed mode. Aliasing prevents accurate measurement of blood velocity. For this reason, continuous-wave Doppler assessment of the ventricular septal defect jet is performed. Continuous-wave Doppler technique allows measurement of velocities of up to 7 m/sec. The beam must be angled until the highest velocity signal is obtained. Both audio and spectral displays are used to achieve optimal signals (Fig. 11.3). Measurement of peak velocities permits the estimation of right ventricular pressure. Peak velocities can be related to interventricular pressure gradients by applying a simplified Bernoulli equation ($\Delta P = 4V^2$).[8] ΔP is the difference in right and left ventricular pressure, and V is the peak velocity across the ventricular septal defect.

In the example shown (Fig. 11.3), a maximal velocity of 4.5 m/sec was recorded across the ventricular septal defect. This value yields a pressure gradient of approximately 80 mm Hg ($4 \times V^2$). Using the systolic blood pressure (105 mm Hg) as the left ventricular pressure, right ventricular systolic pressure can be approximated (105 − 80 = 25 mm Hg).

The direction of the jet across the ventricular septal defect may be quite variable. Therefore, many different transducer positions and angulations should be used to minimize the incident angle

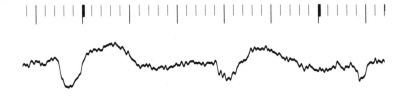

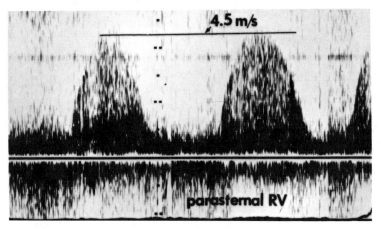

Figure 11.3   Ventricular septal defect. Spectral pattern generated during continuous-wave Doppler examination. The transducer position is paraster-NAL, directed into the right ventricle (RV). A peak velocity of 4.5 m/sec is recorded, resulting in a calculated pressure drop from the left ventricle to the right ventricle of approximately 80 mm Hg.

between the ultrasound beam and the jet. A high-velocity signal indicates a large LV-RV systolic gradient and therefore a lower right ventricular pressure. However, a low-velocity signal may reflect either elevated right ventricular systolic pressure or an inadequate examination caused by an excessive angle between the ultrasound beam and the jet.

Color-coded multigated Doppler imaging has allowed easier detection and localization of ventricular septal defects.[9] This technique has been used to assess the pulmonary arterial pressure

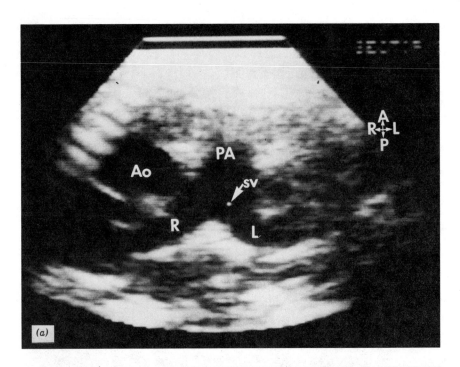

(a)

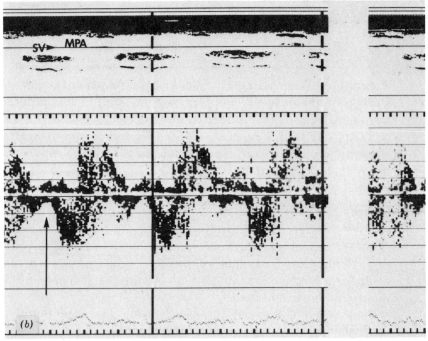

(b)

indirectly by observing the presence or absence of right-to-left shunting.[10] Attempts to quantitate shunt volume are underway. These measurements have not yet been clinically validated.

PATENT DUCTUS ARTERIOSUS

Patent ductus arteriosus can be detected using a two-dimensional echo-guided Doppler examination. Stevenson and co-workers[11] have reported a sensitivity of 96% and a specificity of 100% in a series of 110 patients. With the transducer positioned in the parasternal short-axis position, images of the main pulmonary artery and proximal left and right branches are obtained. Further superior angulation may allow direct visualization of the ductus. By placing the pulsed Doppler sample volume in the distal main pulmonary artery near the origin of the left pulmonary artery, a characteristic audio and spectral signal of the patent ductus arteriosus is recorded. The audio signal registers a continuous flow disturbance, and the spectral signal consists of a diagnostic continuous, high-velocity retrograde flow toward the pulmonary valve (a positive Doppler reflection) alternating with a negative systolic flow (Fig. 11.4). Flow is most turbulent and noticeable in

←

Figure 11.4 Patent ductus arteriosus. (*a*) *Left:* High parasternal two-dimensional echocardiographic short-axis view of the pulmonary bifurcation. The sample volume (SV) is positioned at the pulmonary bifurcation just above the origin of the left (L) pulmonary artery (PA). R, right pulmonary artery; Ao, aorta; A, anterior; L, left; P, posterior; R, right. (*b*) *Right:* With the SV in the main pulmonary artery (MPA), an alternating positively and negatively directed continuous spectral signal, characteristic of patent ductus arteriosus, is recorded. During systole (arrow) blood flow is directed away from the transducer, whereas during diastole flow is toward the transducer. The to-and-fro spectral output is accompanied by a characteristic audible signal.

diastole. Although brief retrograde flow has been seen in other cardiac lesions, the velocity and duration of retrograde flow are much more pronounced in patients with patent ductus arteriosus.[12] From angiographic studies, diastolic ductal flow is known to be abbreviated in patients with elevated pulmonary arterial pressure. A similar abbreviation in diastolic ductal flow has been reported by Doppler investigation in these patients.[13]

A pulsed Doppler examination results in frequency aliasing. Thus, continuous-wave Doppler technique is necessary to assess the aortic-pulmonary pressure gradient (Fig. 11.5). Measurement

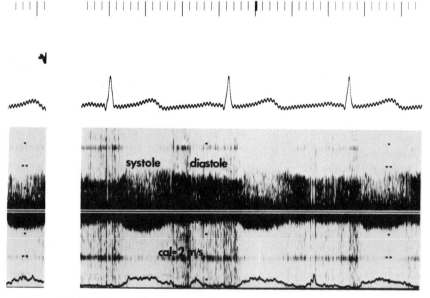

Figure 11.5 Patent ductus arteriosus. The continuous-wave Doppler pattern of patent ductus arteriosus is characterized by an audible, continuous signal as well as a systolic and diastolic spectral disturbance. The systolic component is more prominent than the diastolic one. In the example shown (recorded from the suprasternal notch), the peak velocity is approximately 4 m/sec. This velocity results in a calculated gradient from the aorta to the pulmonary artery of approximately 64 mm Hg. Each calibration mark equals 2 m/sec.

of the velocity in the pulmonary artery can be used to estimate pulmonary artery pressure. In the continuous-wave mode, the transducer is angled to elicit the highest velocity signal. An aortic-pulmonary gradient may be derived from this record. As in patients with ventricular septal defect, high-velocity flow indicates a large pressure gradient and therefore a lower pulmonary artery pressure. A low-velocity signal may indicate either pulmonary hypertension or a large angle between the jet and the Doppler beam.

In the example presented (Fig. 11.5), mean ductal velocity was 4 m/sec. The calculated aortic-pulmonary gradient was 64 mm/Hg ($4 \times V^2$). If the systolic blood pressure is known, an approximation of pulmonary artery pressure can be made (blood pressure − gradient = pulmonary artery pressure).

PULMONARY STENOSIS

The two-dimensional echocardiographic examination of a stenotic pulmonary valve is best performed from the parasternal and subcostal transducer positions. Those imaging planes that best demonstrate the long axis of the pulmonary valve and main pulmonary artery are used for the Doppler examination. In valvar pulmonary stenosis, the Doppler technique permits diagnosis as well as quantification of severity. Normal pulmonary arterial flow is laminar and low in velocity (approximately 1 m/sec).[8] Obstruction to pulmonary flow produces a pressure gradient and increased velocities across the valve. Pulsed Doppler is sensitive in detecting stenosis.[14] However, limitation in velocity measurement prevents quantification of all but the mildest stenoses (Fig. 11.6). Therefore, continuous-wave Doppler is used to estimate severity. The Doppler beam is angled to record the highest-velocity systolic jet across the pulmonary valve (Fig. 11.7). In most cases, the jet is directed away from the transducer position and the spectral signal is displayed below the velocity baseline. As with other stenotic lesions, the Bernoulli equation is used to relate the jet velocity to the pressure gradient.[15]

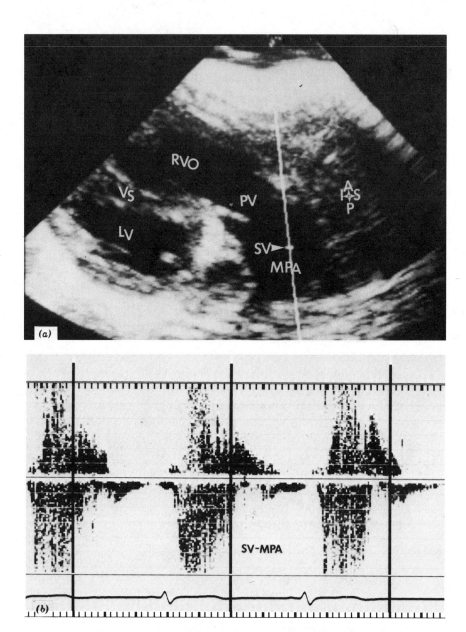

Figure 11.6   Pulmonary stenosis. (*a*) Left: Two-dimensional echocardiographic parasternal right ventricular long-axis view. The right ventricular outflow (RVO), pulmonary valve (PV), and main

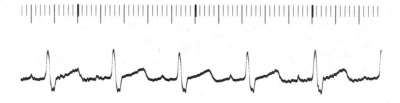

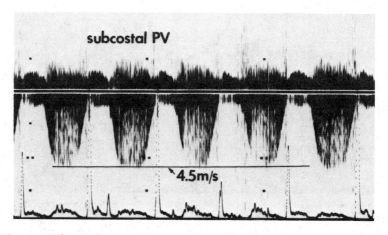

Figure 11.7 Pulmonary stenosis. Continuous wave Doppler spectral pattern of pulmonary stenosis. The transducer position is subcostal, directed toward the pulmonary valve (PV). The peak velocity is approximately 4.5 m/sec. This velocity results in an estimated gradient across the pulmonary valve of 81 mm Hg.

pulmonary artery (MPA) are visualized. The sample volume (SV) is placed within the MPA. LV, left ventricle; VS, ventricular septum; P, posterior, I, inferior; A, anterior; S, superior. (*b*) *Right:* Pulsed doppler spectral pattern of pulmonary stenosis. The SV is placed within the MPA. With each systole, there is a "turbulent" flow disturbance within the MPA characteristic of pulmonary stenosis. There is an accompanying high-pitched audible signal.

125

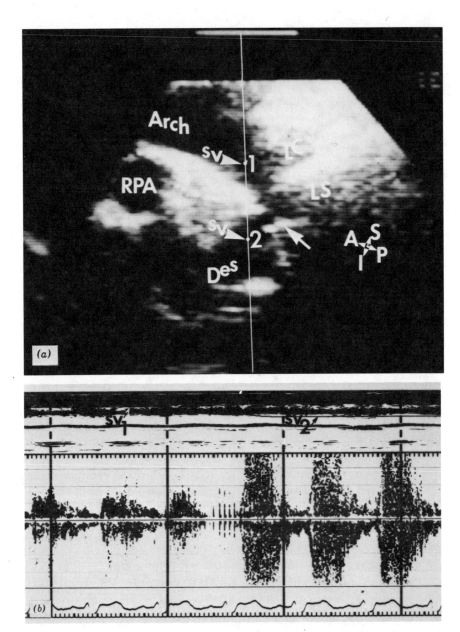

Figure 11.8 Coarctation of the aorta. (a) *Left:* Suprasternal two-dimensional echocardiogram with visualization of suspected coarctation of the aorta (arrow). The coarctation is just distal to the left subclavian artern (LS). Two sample volumes are illustrated, the

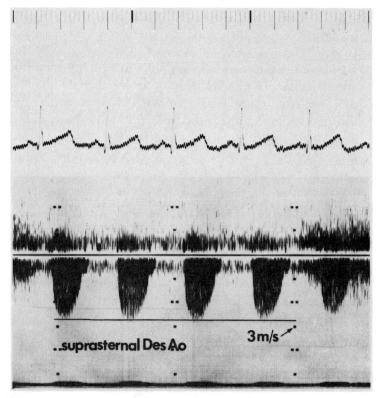

Figure 11.9 Coarctation of the aorta. Continuous-wave Doppler spectral pattern recorded across a coarctation of the aorta. The transducer is positioned in the suprasternal notch directed down the descending thoracic aorta (DesAO). A peak velocity of 2.8 m/sec is recorded. From this value, a gradient of approximately 30 mm Hg is calculated.

first (SV$_1$) above the coarctation and the second (SV$_2$) below it in the descending aorta (DES). RP, right pulmonary artery; ARCH, aortic arch; LC, left carotid; A, anterior; P, posterior; S, superior; I, inferior, (*b*) *Right:* Pulsed Doppler spectral output moving the sample volume located above the coarctation (SV$_1$) below the coarctation. Note the marked change in the systolic flow pattern between the two sampling sites. The increased "turbulence" and aliasing are secondary to increased velocities across the coarctation.

127

In the case example (Fig. 11.7), the peak velocity is 4.5 m/sec. Using the Bernoulli formula, the pressure gradient is 81 mm Hg ($4 \times V^2$).

In children and patients with pulmonary stenosis and poststenotic dilatation of the pulmonary artery, signals are often best recorded from the suprasternal notch or from the left supraclavicular fossa. From these approaches, the high-velocity jet is directed toward the transducer, and therefore the velocity profile is displayed above the baseline.

COARCTATION OF THE AORTA

The two-dimensional echocardiographic diagnosis of coarctation of the aorta is established by imaging from the suprasternal notch, with visualization of the arch and the upper descending thoracic aorta in the long axis. With the pulsed Doppler technique, an abrupt change in the audio signal can be appreciated as the sample volume is moved from the proximal to the distal segments of the descending aorta across the coarctation (Fig. 11.8). The flow profile is high in velocity, systolic, and directed away from the transducer. By placing the transducer in the continuous-wave mode, the pressure gradient across the coarctation can be estimated (Fig. 11.9).

In the example (Fig. 11.9), the peak velocity is 2.8 m/sec and the pressure gradient is approximately 30 mm Hg ($4 \times V^2$). As discussed previously, a low-velocity jet may indicate either a small gradient or a large angle between the jet and the Doppler beam.

CONCLUSION

Doppler echocardiography in both the pulsed and continuous-wave modes plays an important complementary role in a complete two-dimensional echocardiographic examination of patients with congenital heart disease. Not only does this technique allow detection and/or confirmation of intra- and extracardiac shunts, it is very promising in the noninvasive determination of intracardiac and intravascular pressures, pressure gradients, and shunt volumes.

REFERENCES

1. Shub C, Dimopoulos IN, Seward JB, et al: Sensitivity of two-dimensional echocardiography: The direct visualization of atrial septal defect utilizing the subcostal approach: Experience with 154 patients. *J Am Coll Cardiol* 2:127, 1983.

2. Weyman AE, Wann LS, Caldwell RL, et al: Negative contrast echocardiography: A new method for detecting left-to-right shunts. *Circulation* 59:498, 1978.

3. Goldberg SJ, Areias JC, Spitaels SEC, et al: Use of time interval histographic output from echo-Doppler to detect left-to-right atrial shunts. *Circulation* 58:147, 1978.

4. Veyrat C, Abitbol G, Berkman M, et al: Diagnostique et évaluation par écho-Doppler pulsé des insuffisances tricuspidiennes et des communications interventriculaires et interauriculaires. Etude vélocimétrique des shunts. *Arch Mal Coeur* 73:1037, 1980.

5. Kalmanson D, Veyrat C, Derai C, et al: Noninvasive technique for diagnosing atrial septal defect and assessing shunt volume using directional Doppler ultrasound—Correlation with phasic flow velocity patterns of the shunt. *Br Heart J* 34:980, 1972.

6. Goldberg SJ, Sahn DJ, Aver HD, et al: Evaluation of pulmonary and systemic blood flow by two-dimensional Doppler echocardiography using fast Fourier transform spectral analysis. *Am J Cardiol* 50:1394, 1982.

7. Coló J, Stevenson JG, Pearlman AS: A comparison of two-dimensional echocardiography and pulsed Doppler echocardiography for diagnosis of ventricular septal defect. *Circulation* 66:II–232, 1982 (abstracted).

8. Hatle L, Angelsen B: *Doppler Ultrasound in Cardiology*. Philadelphia, Lea & Febiger, 1982.

9. Stevenson JG, Bradestini M, Weiler T, et al: Digital multigate Doppler with color echo and Doppler display—Diagnosis of atrial and ventricular septal defects. *Circulation* 59:II–205, 1979 (abstracted).

10. Stevenson JG, Kawabori I: Color-coded Doppler visualization of flow within ventricular septal defects: Implications for peak pulmonary artery pressure. *Am J Cardiol* 49:944, 1982 (abstracted).

11. Stevenson JG, Kawabori I, Guntheroth WG: Pulsed Doppler echocardiographic diagnosis of patent ductus arteriosus: Sensivity, specificity limitations, and technical features. *Cathet Cardiovasc Diagn* 6:255, 1980.

12. Sahn DJ, Barron JV, Goldberg SJ, et al: Specific two-dimensional echo Doppler criteria for detecting patent ductus arteriosus. *J Am Coll Cardiol* 1:682, 1983 (abstracted).

13. Stevenson JG, Kawabori I, Guntheroth WG: Noninvasive detection of pulmonary hypertension in patent ductus arteriosus by pulsed Doppler echocardiography, *Circulation* 60:355, 1979.

14. Goldberg SJ, Areias JC, Spitaels SEC, et al: Echo Doppler detection of pulmonary stenosis by time-interval histogram analysis. *J Clin Ultrasound* 7:183, 1979.

15. Lima CD, Sahn DJ, Valdes-Cruz LM, et al: Noninvasive prediction of transvalvular pressure gradient in patients with pulmonary stenosis by quantitative two-dimensional echocardiographic Doppler studies. *Circulation* 67:866, 1983.

BIBLIOGRAPHY

Abbasi AS, Allen MW, DeCristofaro D, et al: Detection and estimation of the degree of mitral regurgitation by range-gated pulsed Doppler echocardiography. *Circulation* 61:143, 1980.

Areias JC, Goldberg SJ, Spitaels SEC, et al: An evaluation of range gated pulsed Doppler echocardiography for detecting pulmonary outflow tract obstruction in d-transposition of the great vessels. *Am Heart J* 96:467, 1978.

Baker DW, Rubenstein SA, Lorch GS: Pulsed Doppler echocardiography: Principles and applications. *Am J Med* 63:69, 1977.

Bommer WJ, Mapes R, Miller L, et al: Quantitation of aortic regurgitation with two-dimensional Doppler echocardiography. *Am J Cardiol* 47:412, 1981 (abstracted).

Boughner DR: Assessment of aortic insufficiency by transcutaneous Doppler ultrasound. *Circulation* 52:874, 1975.

Boughner DR, Schuld RL, Persaud JA: Hypertrophic obstructive cardiomyopathy: Assessment by echocardiographic and Doppler ultrasound techniques. *Br Heart J* 37:917, 1975.

Buchtal A, Hanson GC, Peisach AR: Transcutaneous aortovelography. Potentially useful technique in management of critically ill patients. *Br Heart J* 38:451, 1976.

Burckhardt CB: Comparison between spectrum and time interval histogram of ultrasound Doppler signals. *Ultrasound Med Biol* 7:79, 1981.

Ciobanu M, Abbasi AS, Allen M, et al: Pulsed Doppler echocardiography in the diagnosis and estimation of severity of aortic insufficiency. *Am J Cardiol* 49:339, 1982.

Diebold B, Peronneau P, Blanchard D, et al: Non-invasive quantification of aortic regurgitation by Doppler echocardiography. *Br Heart J* 49:167, 1983.

Fantini F, Magherini A: Detection of tricuspid regurgitation with pulsed Doppler echocardiography, in Lancee CT (ed): *Echocardiology: Proceedings of the Third Symposium on Echocardiology*. Rotterdam, the Hague: Martinus Nijhoff Hague, 1979 p 233.

Fisher DC, Sahn DJ, Friedman MJ, et al: The mitral valve orifice method for non-invasive two-dimensional echo Doppler determinations of cardiac output. *Circulation* 67:872, 1983.

Franklin DL, Schlegal WA, Rushmer RF: Blood flow measured by Doppler frequency shift of backscattered ultrasound. *Science* 134:564–565, 1961.

Goldberg S, Areias JC, Spitaels SEC, et al: Echo Doppler detection of pulmonary stenosis by time interval histogram analysis. *J Clin Ultrasound* 7:183, 1979.

Gracia-Derado D, Falzgraf S, Almazan A, et al: Diagnosis of functional tricuspid insufficiency by pulsed wave Doppler ultrasound. *Circulation* 66:1315, 1982.

Hatle L: Non-invasive assessment and differentiation of left ventricular outflow obstruction with Doppler ultrasound. *Circulation* 64:381, 1981.

Hatle L, Angelsen B: *Doppler Ultrasound in Cardiology.* Philadelphia: Lea & Febiger, 1982.

Hatle L, Angelsen B, Tromsdal A: Non-invasive assessment of atrioventricular pressure half time by Doppler ultrasound. *Circulation* 60:1096, 1979.

Hatle L, Angelsen BA, Tromsdal A: Non-invasive assessment of aortic stenosis by Doppler ultrasound. *Br Heart J* 43:284, 1980.

Hatle L, Brubakk A, Tromsdal A, et al: Non-invasive assessment of pressure drop in mitral stenosis by Doppler ultrasound. *Br Heart J* 40:131, 1978.

Hocks APG, Reneman RS, Ruissen CJ, et al: Possibilities and limitations of pulsed Doppler systems, in Lancee CT (ed): *Echocardiology: Proceedings of the Third Symposium on Echocardiology.* Rotterdam, Martinus Nijhoff Hague, 1979, p 413.

Holen J, Aaslid R, Landmark K, et al: Determination of pressure gradient in mitral stenosis with a noninvasive ultrasound Doppler technique. *Acta Med Scand* 199:455, 1976.

Holen J, Aaslid R, Landmark K, et al: Determination of effective orifice area in mitral stenosis from noninvasive ultrasound Doppler data and mitral flow rate. *Acta Med Scand* 201:83, 1977.

Holen J, Simonsen S: Determination of pressure gradient in mitral stenosis with Doppler echocardiography. *Br Heart J* 41:529, 1979.

Huntsman LL, Gams E, Johnson CC, et al: Transcutaneous determinations of aortic blood flow velocities in man. *Am Heart J* 89:605, 1975.

Kalmanson D, Veyrat C, Bouchareine F, et al: Non-invasive recording of mitral valve flow velocity patterns using pulsed Doppler echocardiography. Application to diagnosis and evaluation of mitral valve disease. *Br Heart J* 39:517, 1977.

Kinoshita N, Nimura Y, Okamoto M, et al: Mitral regurgitation in hypertrophic cardiomyopathy. Non-invasive study by two-dimensional Doppler echocardiography. *Br Heart J* 49:574, 1983.

Kitabatake A, Masuyama T, Asao M, et al: Hemodynamic correlates of pulmonary valve motion in man. *Circulation* 68 (suppl 3):332(abstr), 1983.

Lewis J, Kno L, Nelson J, et al: Pulsed Doppler echocardiographic determination of stroke volume and cardiac output from two dimensional apical views: Clinical validation of two new methods. *Circulation* 68(suppl 3):229, 1983.

Libanoff AL, Rodbard S: Evaluation of the severity of mitral stenosis and regurgitation. *Circulation* 33:218, 1966.

Libanoff AL, Rodbard S: Atrioventricular pressure half-time. Measurement of mitral valve orifice area. *Circulation* 38:144, 1968.

Lima CO, Sahn DJ, Valden-Cruz LM, et al: Non-invasive prediction of transvalvar pressure gradient in patients with pulmonary stenosis by quantitative two-dimensional echocardiographic Doppler studies. *Circulation* 67:806, 1983.

Loeber CP, Goldberg SJ, Allen HD: Correlation of Doppler measured ascending aortic, pulmonary, mitral and tricuspid flows. *Circulation* 68(suppl 3):276, 1983.

Lorch G, Rubenstein SA, Baker DW, et al: Doppler echocardiography: Use of a graphical display system. *Circulation* 56:576, 1977.

Mahan G, Dabastani A, Gardin J, et al: Estimation of pulmonary artery pressure by pulsed Doppler echocardiography. *Circulation* 68(suppl 2):367, 1983.

Meijboom EJ, Valdes-Cruz LM, Horowitz S, et al: A two-dimensional Doppler echocardiographic method for calculation of pulmonary and systemic blood flow in a canine model with a variable-sized left-to-right extracardiac shunt. *Circulation* 68:437, 1983.

Meijboom E, Valdes-Cruz LM, Sahn DJ, et al: Echo Doppler method for calculating volume flow across the tricuspid valve: Validation in an open chest canine model and initial clinical studies. *Circulation* 68(suppl 3):331, 1983.

Miyatake K, Kinoshita N, Nagata S, et al: Intracardiac flow pattern in mitral regurgitation studied with combined use of the ultrasonic pulsed Doppler technique and cross-sectional echocardiography. *Am J Cardiol* 45:155, 1980.

Miyatake K, Nimura Y, Sakakibara H, et al: Localization and direction of mitral regurgitant flow in mitral orifice studied with combined use of ultrasonic pulsed Doppler technique and two-dimensional echocardiography. *Br Heart J* 48:449, 1982.

Miyatake K, Okamoto M, Kinoshita N, et al: Pulmonary regurgitation studied with the ultrasonic pulsed Doppler technique. *Circulation* 65:969, 1982.

Miyatake I, Okamoto M, Kinoshita N, et al: Evaluation of tricuspid regurgitation by pulsed Doppler and two dimensional echocardiography. *Circulation* 66:777, 1982.

Murgo JP, Alter BR, Derelky JF, et al: Dynamics of left ventricular ejection in obstructive and nonobstructive hypertrophic cardiomyopathy. *J Clin Invest* 66:1309, 1980.

Patel AK, Rowe GG, Thomsen LA, et al: Detection and estimation of rheumatic mitral regurgitation in the presence of mitral stenosis by pulsed Doppler echocardiography. *Am J Cardiol* 51:986, 1983.

Quinones MA, Young JB, Waggoner AD, et al: Assessment of pulsed Doppler echocardiography in detection and quantification of aortic and mitral regurgitation. *Br Heart J* 44:612, 1980.

Richards KL, Cannon SR, Crawford MH, et al: Non-invasive diagnosis of aortic and mitral valve disease with pulsed Doppler spectral analysis. *Am J Cardiol* 51:1122, 1983.

Sequeira RF, Light LH, Cross G, et al: Transcutaneous aortovelography: A quantitative evaluation. *Br Heart J* 38:443, 1976.

Sequeira RF, Watt I: Assessment of aortic regurgitation by transcutaneous aortovelography. *Br Heart J* 39:929, 1977.

Stewart WJ, Palacius I, Jiang L, et al: Doppler measurement of regurgitant fraction in patients with mitral regurgitation: A new quantitative technique. *Circulation* 68(suppl 3):110, 1983.

Stewart WJ, Pandian NG, Jiang L, et al: Comparison of quantitative Doppler measurement of aortic, mitral and pulmonic flow in an experimental model. *Circulation* 68(suppl 3):110, 1983.

Thuillez C, Theroux P, Bouvassa MG, et al: Pulsed Doppler echocardiographic study of mitral stenosis. *Circulation* 61:381, 1980.

Turnstall Pedoe DS, Macpherson PC, Meldrim SJ: Absolute intracardiac blood velocities measured with continuous wave Doppler and a new real-time spectral display, in Lancee CT (ed): *Echocardiology: Proceedings of the Third Symposium on Echocardiology.* Rotterdam, Martinus Nijhoff Hague, 1979, p 77.

Valdes-Cruz LM, Horowitz S, Mesel E, et al: A pulsed Doppler echocardiographic method for calculation of pulmonary and systemic flow: Accuracy in a canine model with ventricular septal defect. *Circulation* 68:597, 1983.

Valdes-Cruz LM, Horowitz S, Sahn DJ, et al: A simplified mitral valve method for 2-D echo Doppler cardiac output. *Circulation* 68(suppl 3):230, 1983.

Ward JM, Baker DW, Rubenstein SA, et al: Detection of aortic insufficiency by pulsed Doppler echocardiography. *J Clin Ultrasound* 5:5, 1977.

Weinstein IR, Marbarger JP, Perez JE: Ultrasonic assessment of the St.

Jude prosthetic valve: M-mode, two-dimensional, and Doppler echocardiography *Circulation* 68:897–905, 1983.

Wilkes HS, Berger M, Gallerstein PE, et al: Left ventricular outflow obstruction after aortic valve replacement: Detection with continuous wave Doppler ultrasound recording. *J Am Coll Cardiol* 1:250, 1983.

Young JB, Quinones MA, Waggoner AD, et al: Diagnosis and quantification of aortic stenosis with pulsed Doppler echocardiography. *Am J Cardiol* 45:987, 1980.

INDEX

MR — ↑ EF. vol overload S/T too late

mS — ↓ EF (LV protected from LVF)

AS — Sudden death. Severity = $\dfrac{Co}{Sq\ Root\ of\ Gradient}$

— Replace valve if Gradient >100

AR — Surgery of Symptomatic LVJ

Afte Load — vasodilate — good for Regurg not Stenosis. (AS)

A/V area — 2-3 cm

m/V " — 4-5 cm